I0479835

CBD: THE NEW MIRACLE ELIXIR?

CBD OIL: PATIENTS' GUIDE TO MEDICAL CANNABIS USAGE

RALPH CHAMBERLIN
RAYNOLDS M.D.

TABLE OF CONTENTS

CBD Oil vs Hemp Oil vs Cannabis Sativa vs Cannabis Oil: A clear description of each, and their uses

Cannabis Sativa

CBD Oil or Hemp Extract- CBD Oil,

Hemp Oil

Cannabis Oil

CHAPTER 1

Brief Introduction

This book has been written primarily for the sole purpose of shedding light to the grey corners that edge the cannabis world, a long stroll to better understand the ultimate derivative of cannabis: CBD (Cannabidiol). More and more people in the health world are turning to CBD for its ultimate anti-inflammatory and anti-anxiety effects, but just as many are confused about the nature of the compound. This book serves as a know-all guide for those who intend to consume or make use of the powerful compound and its extracts.

The beauty of this book is that, it provides the in-depth knowledge that several publications might have omitted about CBD's inception, to its resulting impact in the present world and potential future.

CHAPTER 2

A COMPREHENSIVE HISTORY OF CANNABIS

Undoubtedly, it appears Wall Street has high hopes for the blossoming cannabis industry -- with cannabis stocks rapidly gaining traction. Tilray (TLRY) , the first marijuana IPO in the United States, has been having a heyday in the market, with one of the most astonishing sessions which saw the stock shoot up over 90% before closing lower. And with an estimated valuation of around $24 billion, cannabis is no longer a joke on The Street. As other companies like Coca-Cola work on getting a piece of the pot pie, it seems the wave of approval for cannabis-based companies and IPOs won't be stopped.

But, how did this all start? What is the history of Cannabis, and how did we get here?

8,000+ BCE The use of hemp cord in pottery was identified at an ancient village site dating back over 10,000 years, located in the area of modern day Taiwan. Finding hemp use and cultivation in this date range puts it as one of the first and oldest known human agriculture crops. As explained by Richard Hamilton in the 2009 Scientific American article on sustainable agriculture "Modern humans emerged some 250,000 years ago, yet agriculture is a fairly recent invention, only about 10,000 years old ... Agriculture is not natural; it is a human invention. It is also the basis of modern civilization." This point was also touched on by Carl Sagan in 1977 when he proposed the possibility that marijuana may have actually been world's first agricultural crop, leading to the development of civilization itself.

6,000 BCE Cannabis seeds and oil used for food in China.

4,000 BCE Textiles made of hemp are used in China and Turkestan.

2,737 BCE First recorded use of cannabis as medicine by Emperor Shen Neng of China.

2,000-800 BCE Bhang (dried cannabis leaves, seeds and stems) is mentioned in the Hindu sacred text Atharvaveda (Science of Charms) as "Sacred Grass", one of the five sacred plants of India. It is used by medicinally and ritually as an offering to Shiva.

1,500 BCE Cannabis cultivated in China for food and fiber. Scythians cultivate cannabis and use it to weave fine hemp cloth.

700-600 BCE The Zoroastrian Zendavesta, an ancient Persian religious text of several hundred volumes refers to bhang as the "good narcotic."

600 BCE HEMP ROPE APPEARS IN SOUTHERN RUSSIA.

700-300 BCE Scythian tribes leave Cannabis seeds as offerings in royal tombs.

500 BCE Scythian couple die and are buried with two small tents covering containers for burning incense. Attached to one tent stick was a decorated leather pouch containing wild Cannabis seeds. This closely matches the stories told by Herodotus. The gravesite, discovered in the late 1940s, was in Pazryk, northwest of the Tien Shan Mountains in modern-day Khazakstan. Hemp is introduced into Northern Europe by the Scythians. An urn containing leaves and seeds of the Cannabis plant, unearthed near Berlin, is found and dated to about this time. Use of hemp products spread throughout northern Europe.

430 BCE Herodotus reports on both ritual and recreation use of Cannabis by the Scythians (Herodotus The Histories 430 B.C. trans. G. Rawlinson).

200 BCE Hemp rope appears in Greece. Chinese Book of Rites mentions hemp fabric.

100 BCE First evidence of hemp paper, invented in China.

100-0 BCE The psychotropic properties of Cannabis are mentioned in the newly compiled herbal Pen Ts'ao Ching.

0-100 CE Construction of Samaritan gold and glass paste stash box for storing hashish, coriander, or salt, buried in Siberian tomb.

23-79 Pliny the Elder's The Natural History mentions hemp rope and marijuana's analgesic effects.

47-127 Plutarch mentions Thracians using cannabis as an intoxicant.

70 Dioscorides, a physician in Nero's army, lists medical marijuana in his Pharmacopoeia.

100 IMPORTED HEMP ROPE APPEARS IN ENGLAND.

105 Legend suggests that Ts'ai Lun invents hemp paper in China, 200 years after its actual appearance (see 100 BCE above).

130-200 Greek physician Galen prescribes medical marijuana.

200 First pharmacopoeia of the East lists medical marijuana. Chinese surgeon Hua T'o uses marijuana as an anesthetic.

300 A young woman in Jerusalem receives medical marijuana during childbirth.

570 The French queen Arnegunde is buried with hemp cloth.

500-600 The Jewish Talmud mentions the euphoriant properties of Cannabis.

850 VIKINGS TAKE HEMP ROPE AND SEEDS TO ICELAND.

900 Arabs learn techniques for making hemp paper.

900-1000 Scholars debate the pros and cons of eating hashish. Use spreads throughout Arabia.

1000 Hemp ropes appear on Italian ships. Arabic physician Ibn Wahshiyah's On Poisons warns of marijuana's potential dangers.

1090-1124 In Khorasan, Persia, Hasan ibn al-Sabbah, recruits followers to commit assassinations...legends develop around their supposed use of hashish. These legends are some of the earliest written tales of the discovery of the inebriating powers of Cannabis and the use of Hashish by a paramilitary organization as a hypnotic (see U.S. military use, 1942 below). Early 12th Century Hashish smoking becomes very popular throughout the Middle East.

1155-1221 Persian legend of the Sufi master Sheik Haydar's personal discovery of Cannabis and his own alleged invention of hashish with it's subsequent spread to Iraq, Bahrain, Egypt and Syria. Another of the ealiest written narratives of the use of

Cannabis as an inebriant.

1171-1341 During the Ayyubid dynasty of Egypt, Cannabis is introduced by mystic devotees from Syria.

1200 1,001 Nights, an Arabian collection of tales, describes hashish's intoxicating and aphrodisiac properties.

13th Century The oldest monograph on hashish, Zahr al-'arish fi tahrim al-hashish, was written. It has since been lost. Ibn al-Baytar of Spain provides a description of the psychoactive nature of Cannabis. Arab traders bring Cannabis to the Mozambique coast of Africa.

1271-1295 Journeys of Marco Polo in which he gives second-hand reports of the story of Hasan ibn al-Sabbah and his "assassins" using hashish. First time reports of Cannabis have been brought to the attention of Europe.

1300 Ethiopian pipes containing marijuana suggest the herb has spread from Egypt to the rest of Africa.

1378 Ottoman Emir Soudoun Scheikhouni issues one of the first edicts against the eating of hashish.

1526 Babur Nama, first emperor and founder of Mughal Empire learned of hashish in Afghanistan.

1532 French physician Rabelais's gargantua and Pantagruel mentions marijuana's medicinal effects.

1533 King Henry VIII fines farmers if they do not raise hemp for industrial use.

1549 Angolan slaves brought cannabis with them to the sugar plantations of northeastern Brazil. They were permitted to plant their cannabis between rows of cane, and to smoke it between harvests.

1550 The epic poem, Benk u Bode, by the poet Mohammed Ebn Soleiman Foruli of Baghdad, deals allegorically with a dialectical battle between wine and hashish.

1563 Portuguese physician Garcia da Orta reports on marijuana's medicinal effects.

1578 China's Li Shih-Chen writes of the antibiotic and anti-emetic effects of marijuana.

1600 ENGLAND BEGINS TO IMPORT HEMP FROM RUSSIA.

1606-1632 French and British cultivate Cannabis for hemp at their colonies in Port Royal (1606), Virginia (1611), and Plymouth (1632).

1616 Jamestown settlers began growing the hemp plant for its unusually strong fiber and used it to make rope, sails, and clothing.

1621 Burton's Anatomy of Melancholy suggests marijuana may treat depression.

1600-1700 Use of hashish, alcohol, and opium spreads among the population of occupied Constantinople. Hashish becomes a major trade item between Central Asia and South Asia.

1753 LINNAEUS CLASSIFIES CANNABIS SATIVA.

1764 Medical marijuana appears in The New England Dispensatory.

1776 KENTUCKY BEGINS GROWING HEMP.

1794 Medical marijuana appears in The Edinburgh New Dispensary.

1798 Napoleon discovers that much of the Egyptian lower class habitually uses hashish. Soldiers returning to France bring the tradition with them, and he declares a total prohibition.

1800 Marijuana plantations flourished in Mississippi, Georgia, California, South Carolina, Nebraska, New York, and Kentucky. Also during this period, smoking hashish was popular throughout France and to a lesser degree in the US. Hashish production expands from Russian Turkestan into Yarkand in Chinese Turkestan.

1809 Antoine Sylvestre de Sacy, a leading Arabist, suggests a base etymology between the words "assassin" and "hashishin" -- subsequent linguest study disproves his theory.

1840 In America, medicinal preparations with a Cannabis base are available. Hashish is available in Persian pharmacies.

1842 Irish physician O'Shaughnessy publishes cannabis research in English medical journals.

1843 French author Gautier publishes The Hashish Club.

1846 FRENCH PHYSICIAN MOREAU PUBLISHES HASHISH AND MENTAL ILLNESS

1850 Cannabis is added to The U.S. Pharmacopoeia.

1850-1915 Marijuana was widely used throughout United States as a medicinal drug and could easily be purchased in pharmacies and general stores.

1854 Whittier writes the first American work to mention cannabis as an intoxicant.

1856 British tax "ganja" and "charas" trade in India.

1857 American writer Ludlow publishes The Hasheesh Eater.

1858 French poet Baudelaire publishes On the Artificial Ideal.

1870-1880 First reports of hashish smoking on the Greek mainland.

1890 Greek Department of Interior prohibits importance,

cultivation and use of hashish. Hashish is made illegal in Turkey. Sir J.R. Reynolds, chief physician to Queen Victoria, prescribes medical marijuana to her.

1893-1894 The India Hemp Drugs Commission Report is issued. 70,000 to 80,000 kg per year of hashish is legally imported into India from Central Asia.

1906 In the U.S. the Pure Food and Drug Act is passed, regulating the labeling of products containing Alcohol, Opiates, Cocaine, and Cannabis, among others.

Early 20th Century Hashish smoking remains very popular throughout the Middle East.

1910 The Mexican Revolution caused an influx of Mexican immigrants who introduced the habit of recreational use (instead of it's generally medicinal use) into American society.

1914 The Harrison Act in the U.S. defined use of Marijuana (among other drugs) as a crime.

1916 United States Department of Agriculture (USDA) chief scientists Jason L. Merrill and Lyster H. Dewey created paper made from hemp pulp, which they concluded was "favorable in comparison with those used with pulp wood" in USDA Bulletin No. 404. From the book "The Emperor Wears No Clothes" by Jack Herer the USDA Bulletin N. 404 reported that one acre of hemp, in annual rotation over a 20-year period, would produce as much pulp for paper as 4.1 acres (17,000 m2) of trees being cut down over the same 20-year period. This process would use only 1/7 to 1/4 as much polluting sulfur-based acid chemicals to break down the glue-like lignin that binds the fibers of the pulp, or even none at all using soda ash. The problem of dioxin contamination of rivers is avoided in the hemp paper making process, which does not need to use chlorine bleach (as the wood pulp paper making process requires) but instead safely substitutes hydrogen peroxide in the bleaching process. ... If the new (1916) hemp pulp paper process were legal today, it would soon replace about 70% of all wood pulp paper, including computer printout paper, corrugated boxes and paper bags. However, mass production of cheap news print from hemp had not developed in any country, and hemp was a relatively easy target because factories already had made large investments in equipment to handle cotton, wool, and linen, but there were relatively small investments in hemp production.

1915-1927 In the U.S. cannabis begins to be prohibited for nonmedical use. Prohibition first begins in California (1915), followed by Texas (1919), Louisiana (1924), and New York (1927).

1919 The 18th Amendment to the U.S. Constitution banned the manufacture, sale, and transportation of alcohol and positioned marijuana as an attractive alternative leading to an increase in use of the substance.

1920s Greek dictator Ioannis Metaxas cracks down on hashish smoking. Hashish smuggled into Egypt from Greece, Syria, Lebanon, Turkey, and Central Asia.

1924 Russian botanists classify another major strain of the plant, Cannabis ruderalis.

1926 LEBANESE HASHISH PRODUCTION IS PROHIBITED.

1928 Recreational use of Cannabis is banned in Britain.

1930 The Yarkand region of Chinese Turkestan exports 91,471 kg of hashish legally into the Northwest Frontier and Punjab regions of India. Legal taxed imports of hashish continue into India from Central Asia.

1933 The U.S. congress repealed the 21st Amendment, ending alcohol prohibition; 4 years later the prohibition of marijuana will be in full effect.

1934-1935 Chinese government moves to end all Cannabis cultivation in Yarkand and charas traffic from Yarkand. Hashish production become illegal in Chinese Turkestan.

1936 The American propaganda film Reefer Madness was made to scare American youth away from using Cannabis. American Dollars Spent, and American Citizens Arrested, Because of the Dubious "War On Drugs" THIS Year Alone ...

1937 U.S. Congress passed the Marijuana Tax Act which criminalized the drug. In response Dr. William C. Woodward, testifying on behalf of the AMA, told Congress that, "The American Medical Association knows of no evidence that marijuana is a dangerous drug" and warned that a prohibition "loses sight of the fact that future investigation may show that there are substantial medical uses for Cannabis." His comments were ignored by Congress. A part of the testimony for Congress to pass the 1937 act derived from articles in newspapers owned by William Randolph Hearst, who had significant financial interests in the timber industry, which manufactured his newsprint paper.

1938 Supply of hashish from Chinese Turkestan nearly ceases. The U.S. company DuPont patented the processes for creating plastics from coal and oil and a new process for creating paper from wood pulp.

1940S GREEK HASHISH SMOKING TRADITION FADES.

1941 Cannabis is removed from the U.S. Pharmacopoeia and it's medicinal use is no longer recognized in America. The same year the Indian government considers cultivation in Kashmir to fill void of hashish from Chinese Turkestan. Hand-rubbed charas from Nepal is choicest hashish in India during World War II.

1942 U.S. scientists working at the Office of Strategic Services (OSS), the CIA's wartime predecessor, began to develop a chemical substance that could break down the psychological defenses of enemy spies and POWs. After testing several compounds, the OSS scientists selected a potent extract of marijuana as the best available "truth serum." The cannabis concoction was given the code name TD, meaning Truth Drug. When injected into food or tobacco cigarettes, TD helped loosen the reserve of recalcitrant interrogation subjects.

1945 Legal hashish consumption continues in India. Hashish use in Greece flourishes again.

1951 The Boggs Act and the Narcotics Control Act in the U.S. increases all drug penalties and laid down mandatory sentences.

1960 Czech researchers confirm the antibiotic and analgesic effects of cannabis.

1963 TURKISH POLICE SEIZE 2.5 TONS OF HASHISH.

1965 First reports of the strain Cannibis afghanica and was used for hashish production in northern Afghanistan.

1967 "Smash", the first hashish oil appears. Red Lebanese reaches California.

1970-1972 Huge fields of Cannabis are cultivated for hashish production in Afghanistan. Afghani hashish varieties introduced to North America for sinsemilla production. Westerners bring metal sieve cloths to Afghanistan. Law enforcement efforts against hashish begin in Afghanistan.

1970 The US National Organization for the Reform of Marijuana Laws (NORML) forms. That same year the Comprehensive Drug Abuse Prevention and Control Act repealed mandatory penalties for drug offenses and marijuana was categorized separately from other narcotics.

1971 First evidence suggesting marijuana may help glaucoma patients.

1972 The Nixon-appointed Shafer Commission urged use of cannabis be re-legalized, but their recommendation was ignored. U.S. Medical research picks up pace. Proposition 19 in California to legalize marijuana use is rejected by a voter margin of 66-33%.

1973 Nepal bans the Cannabis shops and charas (hand-rolled hash) export. Afghan government makes hashish production and sales illegal. Afghani harvest is pitifully small.

1975 Nabilone, a cannabinoid-based medication appears.

1976 The U.S. federal government created the Investigational New Drug (IND) Compassionate Use research program to allow patients to receive up to nine pounds of cannabis from the government each year. Today, five surviving patients still receive medical cannabis from the federal government, paid for by federal tax dollars. At the same time the U.S. FDA continues to list marijuana as Schedule I meaning: "A high potential for abuse with no accepted medical value."

1977 Carl Sagan proposes that marijuana may have been the world's first agricultural crop, leading to the development of civilization itself: "It would be wryly interesting if in human history the cultivation of marijuana led generally to the invention of agriculture, and thereby to civilization." Carl Sagan, The Dragons of Eden, Speculations on the Origin of Human Intelligence p 191 footnote.

1977-1981 U.S. President Carter, including his assistant for drug policy, Dr. Peter Bourne, pushed for decriminalization of marijuana, with the president himself asking Congress to abolish federal criminal penalties for those caught with less than one ounce of marijuana.

1980s Morocco becomes one of, if not the largest, hashish producing and exporting nations. "Border hashish" is produced in northwestern Pakistan along the Afghan border to avoid Soviet-Afghan war.

1985 Hashish is still produced by Muslims of Kashgar and Yarkland in Northwest China. In the U.S. the FDA approves dronabinol, a synthetic THC, for cancer patients.

1986 President Reagan signed the Anti-Drug Abuse Act, reinstating mandatory minimums and raising federal penalties for possession and distribution and officially begins the U.S. international "war on drugs."

1987 Moroccan government cracks down upon Cannabis cultivation in lower elevations of the Rif Mountains.

1988 U.S. DEA administrative law Judge Francis Young finds, after thorough hearings, that marijuana has a clearly established medical use and should be reclassified as a prescriptive drug. His recommendation is ignored.

1992 In reaction to a surge of requests from AIDS patients for medical marijuana, the U.S. government closes the Compassionate Use program. That same year the pharmaceutical medication dronabinol is approved for AIDS-wasting syndrome.

1993 Cannabis eradication efforts resume in Morocco.

1994 Border hashish still produced in Pakistan. Heavy fighting between rival Muslim clans continues to upset hashish trade in Afghanistan.

1995 Introduction of hashish-making equipment and appearance of locally produced hashish in Amsterdam coffee shops.

1996 California (the first U.S. state to ban marijuana use, see 1915) became the first U.S. State to then re-legalize medical marijuana use for people suffering from AIDS, cancer, and other serious illnesses. A similar bill was passed in Arizona the same year. This was followed by the passage of similar initiatives in Alaska, Colorado, Maine, Montana, Nevada, Oregon, Washington, Washington D.C., Hawaii, Maryland, New Mexico, Rhode Island, and Vermont.

1997 The American Office of National Drug Control Policy commissioned the Institute of Medicine (IOM) to conduct a comprehensive study of the medical efficacy of cannabis therapeutics. The IOM concluded that cannabis is a safe and effective medicine, patients should have access, and the government should expand avenues for research and drug development. The federal government completely ignored its findings and refused to act on its recommendations.

1997-2001 In direct contradiction to the IOM recomendations, President Clinton, continuing the Regan and Bush "war on drugs" era, began a campaign to arrest and prosecute medical cannabis patients and their providers in California and elsewhere.

1999 Hawaii and North Dakota unsuccessfully attempt to legalize hemp farming. The U.S. DEA reclassifies dronabinol as a schedule III drug, making the medication easier to prescribe while marijuana itself continues to be listed Schedule I as having "no accepted medical use."

2000 LEGALIZATION INITIATIVE IN ALASKA FAILS.

2001 Britain's Home Secretary, David Blunkett, proposes relaxing the classification of cannabis from a class B to class C. Canada adopts federal laws in support of medical marijuana, and by 2003 Canada becomes the first country in the world to approve medical marijuana nation-wide.

2001-2009 Under President G.W. Bush the U.S. federal government intensified its "war on drugs" targeting both patients and doctors across the state of California.

2005 Marc Emery, a Canadian citizen and the largest distributor of marijuana seeds into the United States from approximately 1995 through July 2005 was on the FBI #1 wanted drug list for years and was eventually indicted by the U.S. DEA. He was extradited from Canada for trial in the U.S. in May 2010.

2009 President Obama made steps toward ending the very unsuccessful 20-year "war on drugs" initiated during the Regan administration by stating that individual drug use is really a public health issue, and should be treated as such. Under his guidance, the U.S. Justice Department announced that federal prosecutors will no longer pursue medical marijuana users and distributors who comply with state laws.

2010 Marc Emery of Vancouver, BC, Canada, was sentenced on September 10 in a U.S. District Court in Seattle to five years in prison and four years of supervised release for "conspiracy to manufacture marijuana" (eg. selling marijuana seeds).

2010 Proposition 19 to legalize marijuana in California is placed back on the ballet (named The Regulate, Control and Tax Cannabis Act of 2010). Current voter poles suggest that the proposition has about 50% population support and will likely win or loose by a margin of only 2%.

Oct 2010 Just weeks before the November 02 California election on Prop. 19 Attorney General Eric Holder said federal authorities would continue to enforce U.S. laws that declare the drug is illegal, even if voters approve the initiative, stating "we will vigorously enforce the (Controlled Substances Act) against those individuals and organizations that possess, manufacture or distribute marijuana for recreational use."

Nov 2010 California Proposition 19, also known as the Regulate, Control and Tax Cannabis Act of 2010, was narrowly defeated by 53.6% of the vote. This would have legalized various marijuana-related activities in California, allowing local governments to regulate these activities, permitting local governments to impose and collect marijuana-related fees and taxes, and authorizing various criminal and civil penalties.

Nov 2012 The States of Colorado and Washington legalize marijuana / cannabis for recreational use; promises are made to the people that these new initiatives will have no impact on medical marijuana in those states. The country of Uruguay legalizes marijuana / cannabis for recreational use. The US District of Columbia decriminalizes personal use and possession of marijuana / cannabis.

July 07, 2014 Cannabis City becomes Seattle's very first legal marijuana shop for over-the-counter purchase & recreational use. This generated world-wide media attention and a serious discussion over the legalization of marijuana and a possible end to the American "drug war." The first purchase, by Deb Green a 65-year old marathon-running grandmother from Ballard, is part of the collection of the Museum of History and Industry in Seattle, Washington.

Nov 2014 The States of Alaska and Oregon legalize marijuana / cannabis for recreational use; the States of California, Nevada, Arizona, Hawaii and Massachusetts all begin to draft legalization legislation.

July 24, 2015 With the passage of Senate Bill 5052 Washington State medical marijuana comes fully under the control of the newly re-named Washington Liquor and Cannabis Board (LCB).

CHAPTER 3

CBD: THE NEW MIRACLE ELIXIR?

Cannabidiol is being touted as a magical elixir, a cure-all now available in bath bombs, dog treats and even pharmaceuticals. But maybe it's just a fix for our anxious times. It's hard to say the precise moment when CBD, the voguish cannabis derivative, went from being a fidget spinner alternative for stoners to a mainstream panacea.

Maybe it was in January, when Mandy Moore, hours before the Golden Globes, told Coveteur that she was experimenting with CBD oil to relieve the pain from wearing high heels. "It could be a really exciting evening," she said. "I could be floating this year."

Maybe it was in July, when Willie Nelson introduced a line of CBD-infused coffee beans called Willie's Remedy. "It's two of my favorites, together in the perfect combination," he said in a statement.

Or maybe it was earlier this month, when Dr. Sanjay Gupta gave a qualified endorsement of CBD on "The Dr. Oz Show." "I think there is a legitimate medicine here," he said. "We're talking about something that could really help people."

So the question now becomes: Is this the dawning of a new miracle elixir, or does all the hype mean we have already reached Peak CBD?

Either way, it would be hard to script a more of-the-moment salve for a nation on edge. With its proponents claiming that CBD treats ailments as diverse as inflammation, pain, acne, anxiety, insomnia, depression, post-traumatic stress and even cancer, it's easy to wonder if this all natural, non-psychotropic and widely available cousin of marijuana represents a cure for the 21st century itself.

The ice caps are melting, the Dow teeters, and a divided country seems headed for divorce court. Is it any wonder, then, that everyone seems to be reaching for the tincture? With CBD popping up in nearly everything — bath bombs, ice cream, dog treats — it is hard to overstate the speed at which CBD has moved from the Burning Man margins to the cultural center.

A year ago, it was easy to be blissfully unaware of CBD. Now, to measure the hype, it's as if everyone suddenly discovered yoga. Or penicillin. Or maybe oxygen. Even so, you ask, what is CBD? Plenty of people still have no idea. CBD is short for cannabidiol, an abundant chemical in the cannabis plant. Unlike its more famous cannabinoid cousin, THC (tetrahydrocannabinol), CBD does not make you stoned. Which is not to say that you feel utterly normal when you take it.

TRAVEL

As states continue to legalize, you can expect to see cannabis-based edibles on the menu during your next hotel resturant visit. Moreover, you are unlikely to find yourself microwaving frozen burritos at midnight after taking CBD, unlike with cannabis.

"I'm a 30 years old male who has not experienced not one anxiety free day in my grownup life," wrote one user on a CBD forum on a social media platform earlier this month. "Some weeks ago I started taking CBD-oil 10 percent and I can't even describe how amazing I feel. For the first time in 15 years I feel happy and look forward to living a long life." Such testimonials make CBD seem like a perfect cure for our times. Every cultural era, after all, has its defining psychological malady. This also means that every era has its signature drug.

The defining sociological condition today, especially among millennials, is arguably anxiety: anxiety about our political dysfunction, anxiety about terrorism, anxiety about climate change, anxiety about student loan debt, even anxiety about artificial intelligence taking away all the good jobs. The anxiety feels even more acute since the wired generation feels continuously bombarded by new reasons to freak out, thanks to their smart devices.

What a convenient time for Mother Nature to bestow a perma-chillax cure that seems to tie together so many cultural threads at once: our obsession with self-care and wellness, the mainstreaming of alternative therapies and the relentless march of legalized marijuana.

"That seems like our knight in shinning armor," Ms. vonhagen said.

Despite its cannabis origins, CBD is not marketed as a recreational drug, but almost as its opposite: as a corrective to the ill effects of alcohol and even marijuana itself, which makes it catnip for hard-charging professionals who need to be fresh for an early morning breakfast meeting.

Fewer hangovers is also the sales pitch for bars that whip up CBD-infused negronis and old-fashioned cocktails. When added to dishes like shrimp toast, CBD (which is flavorless) can function as a social lubricant, just like a wine pairing, but without, according to proponents, the hangover. But nowhere does the fervor for CBD seem greater than in health and beauty, where cannabidiol is often packaged with buzzy terms like "single origin," "small batch" and "plant based."

Among beauty products alone, CBD has already achieved cliché status, popping up in blemish creams, sleeping masks, shampoos, hair conditioners, eye serums, anti-acne lotions, mascaras, massage oils, soaps, lip balms, bath bombs, anti-wrinkle serums, muscle rubs and a Sephora aisle's worth of moisturizers, face lotions and body creams. Even the bedroom is not safe from the CBD invasion, to judge by the spate of CBD sexual lubricants on shelves.

CBD: HUMBUG OR MIRACLE DRUG?

There's one problem associated with that approach. When people turn to CBD-infused coconut lattes to cure acne and erectile dysfunction, it is not easy to separate hype from science. Skeptics who assume CBD is just 21st-century humbug, however, may be surprised to learn that the substance is being studied as a potential treatment for maladies as diverse as schizophrenia, insomnia and cancer.

The National Institutes of Health database lists about 150 of studies involving CBD as a treatment for conditions as varied as infantile spasms and Parkinson's disease. And the research has led to medical treatments. In June, the Food and Drug Administration approved a cannabidiol-based drug called Epidiolex as a treatment for severe forms of epilepsy, representing the first government-sanctioned medical use for CBD.

Preliminary research also indicates that CBD may be effective as an antipsychotic in reducing the symptoms of schizophrenia, with fewer side effects compared with current antipsychotic drugs.CBD has also shown promise to reduce cravings among people addicted to opioids, according to a study published in Neurotherapeutics. It may fight cancer, too.

That's not to say that a CBD-laced gummy or two should be considered medicine. Don't go chugging a shot of CBD oil just yet. Much of the research is in its infancy, and the purity and dosage of some CBD consumer products may not reliable.

CBD can have negative interactions with many medications, so potential users should talk to their doctors before taking it.

There are legal hazards as well. As with all cannabis products, the federal government categorizes CBD products other than Epidiolex as a Schedule 1 drug, like heroin, according to the Drug Enforcement Administration. And cannabis remains illegal under federal law, even in states that have legalized marijuana for medical or recreational use. Although there have been scattered raids of CBD retailers around the country, several states, including Alabama, Texas, Florida and Oklahoma, have passed laws approving specific CBD products to treat specific ailments. And CBD shops have cropped up nationwide, in Los Angeles, Oklahoma City and Austin, Tex., to name just a few cities.

In New York City, for example, CBD tinctures and other products can be bought at specialty shops, health food stores, yoga studios, flea markets, boutiques and even some corner delis. Aside from a federal crackdown, the only thing that may eventually kill CBD's momentum is hype itself.

The frothy claims about CBD sets up some false expectations that the molecule will never be able to live up to. Not only are questionable claims an invitation for government regulation, but they risk making even legitimate applications seem dubious. In isolation, CBD obviously does have some benefits, but it's certainly not a catchall for all the world's health problems.

CHAPTER 4

Cannabis in the United States

In the United States, early colonists grew hemp (a cannabis plant) often for use in textiles or even things like making rope. By the 1600s, farmers in colonies like Virginia, Massachusetts and Connecticut were growing the plant. It has even been suggested that Thomas Jefferson and George Washington grew hemp on their plantations.

RACIAL STIGMA

During the nineteenth century, the word "cannabis" was almost completely used to refer to the plant. However, once anti-Mexican sentiment in the United States began to rise in the early twentieth century, the term was switched to "marijuana" to draw attention to the drug's use by Mexicans -- and thereby attempt to carry negative connotation.

Some common theories about the racial undertones of the stigma against cannabis circulate around the government associating marijuana use with dangerous, murderous tendencies brought on by "locoweed" -- Mexican cannabis. This stigma, combined with the rising racial tensions against people of color, contributed to increasing federal regulation of the drug.

The political upheaval in United Mexican States country (North American nations) that culminated in the Revolution of 1910 led to a wave of Mexican immigration to states throughout the American Southwest. The prejudices and fears that greeted these peasant immigrants also extended to their ancient suggest that of intoxication: smoking marijuana. Police officers in Texas claimed that marijuana incited violent crimes aroused a 'lust for blood' and gave its users 'superhuman strength.' Rumors spread that Mexicans were distributing this 'killer weed' to unsuspecting American schoolchildren. Sailors and West Indian immigrants brought the practice of smoking marijuana to port cities on the Gulf of Mexico. In New Orleans, newspaper articles associated the drug with African-Americans, jazz musicians, prostitutes, and underworld whites.

'The Marijuana Menace,' as sketched by anti-drug campaigners, was personified by inferior races and social deviants.

Additionally, the infamous quote by Harry Anslinger -- one amongst the leaders of the prohibition -- reads that "There are one hundred thousand total marijuana smokers in the U.S., and most are Negroes, Hispanics, Filipinos, and entertainers. Their Satanic music, jazz and swing result from marijuana use. This marijuana causes white ladies to seek sexual relations with Negroes, entertainers and any others."

While the racial language may have since for the most part dissipated, it was reported that in 2016, 600,000 cannabis-related arrests took place, with the large majority affecting minorities.

MARIJUANA TAX ACT OF 1937

By 1937, the Marijuana Tax Act effectively banned sale of the plant by imposing heavy excise taxes on sale, possession, or transportation of hemp. This act, set by the federal U.S. government, lead to the first marijuana-related arrest in October of 1937 of 58-year-old Samuel Caldwell -- a farmer caught selling cannabis

Although marijuana continued to be grown in the United States, the last official hemp fields were planted in Wisconsin in 1957.The Marijuana Tax Act levied a huge tax so that people would [be] dissuaded from buying cannabis. So, 1941, cannabis was removed from all pharmacopoeias (you couldn't get it in stores and couldn't find any evidence of it.) And since then, there has been stigma.

A BRIEF HISTORY OF THE DRUG WAR

By 1970, the Controlled Substances Act, as part of the "War on Drugs" spearheaded by President Richard Nixon, repealed the Marijuana Tax Act, but classified cannabis as a Schedule 1 drug -- in the same category as heroin, LSD, cocaine and ecstasy. Drugs, according to the administration, were "public enemy number one." Marijuana remains a Schedule 1 drug today, causing great difficulties for those wishing to study its medicinal properties. Contrary to numerous medical opinions, the definition of Schedule 1 seems to clash with marijuana's actual benefits.

Quite a number of people believe in the efficacy [of marijuana], but either they cannot use it because they're associated with universities or hospitals which receive federal grants, so they can't use it, or, they're afraid to use it and have the DEA coming after them because it's still labeled as a controlled substance category 1. Which means, by definition, no medical use and highly addictive.

Still, Nixon's Act largely ignored the National Commission on Marijuana and Drug Abuse's report in 1972 titled "Marijuana: A Signal of Misunderstanding," which prompted lesser penalties for small possessions and incremental prohibition.

THE EARLY STAGES OF DRUG PROHIBITION

Many currently illegal drugs, such as marijuana, opium, coca, and psychedelics have been used for thousands of years for both medical and spiritual purposes. thus why are some medication legal and different drugs illegal today? It's not based on any scientific assessment of the relative risks of these drugs – however it has everything to do with who is associated with these drugs.

The first anti-opium laws in the 1870s were directed at Chinese immigrants. The first anti-cocaine laws in the early 1900s were directed at black men within the South. The 1st anti-marijuana laws, in the geographic area and the Southwest in the 1910s and 20s, were directed at Mexican migrants and Mexican Americans. Today, Latino and particularly black communities square measure still subject to wildly disproportionate drug enforcement and sentencing practices.

NIXON AND THE GENERATION GAP

In the 1960s, as medication became symbols of youthful rebellion, social upheaval, and political dissent, the govt halted scientific research to judge their medical safety and effectualness.

In June 1971, President Nixon declared a "war on drugs." He dramatically redoubled the size and presence of federal drug control agencies, and pushed through measures such as mandatory sentencing and no-knock warrants.

A prime Nixon aide, John Ehrlichman, later admitted: "You want to understand what this was really all about. The President Nixon campaign in 1968, and the Nixon White House at the moment, had two enemies: the antiwar left and black individuals. You understand what I'm saying. We knew we couldn't make it illegal to be either against the war or black, however by getting the public to associate the hippies with marijuana and blacks with hard drug, and then criminalizing both heavily, we tend to could disrupt those communities. we tend to may arrest their leaders, raid their homes, break up their meetings, and vilify them night once night on the evening news. Did we understand we tend to were lying about the drugs? Of course we did." Nixon temporarily placed marijuana in Schedule One, the foremost restrictive category of drugs, unfinished review by a commission he appointed semiconductor diode by Republican Pennsylvania Governor Raymond Shafer.

In 1972, the commission unanimously recommended de-criminalizing the possession and distribution of marijuana for private use. Nixon ignored the report and rejected its recommendations.

Between 1973 and 1977, however, eleven states decriminalized marijuana possession. In January 1977, President Jimmy Carter was inaugurated on a campaign platform that included marijuana decriminalization. In Oct 1977, the Senate Judiciary Committee voted to allow possession of up to an ounce of marijuana for personal use.

Within few years, though, the tide had shifted. Proposals to allow marijuana were abandoned as parents became increasingly involved about high rates of teen marijuana use. Marijuana was ultimately caught up in a broader cultural backlash against the perceived permissiveness of the 1970s.

THE 1980S AND 90S: DRUG HYSTERIA AND INCREASING INCARCERATION RATES

The presidency of the United States marked the start of long amount of skyrocketing rates of incarceration, mostly thanks to his unprecedented expansion of the drug war. The number of people behind bars for nonviolent drug law offenses magnified from 50,000 in 1980 to over 400,000 by 1997.

Public concern about illicit drug use engineered throughout the 1980s, mostly due to media portrayals of people addicted to the smokeable form of cocaine dubbed "crack." presently when Ronald Reagan took workplace in 1981, his wife, Nancy Reagan, began a highly-publicized anti-drug campaign, coining the saying "Just Say No." This set the stage for the zero tolerance policies implemented in the mid-to-late Eighties. Los Angeles police captain Daryl Gates, United Nations agency believed that "casual drug users ought to be taken out and shot," supported the DARE drug education program, which was quickly adopted nationwide despite the shortage of proof of its effectiveness. The increasingly harsh drug policies also blocked the expansion of syringe access programs and alternative hurt reduction policies to scale back the speedy spread of HIV/AIDS.

In the late Eighties, a political hysteria about medicine led to the passage of lawmaker penalties in Congress and state legislatures that rapidly increased the prison population. In 1985, the proportion of Americans polled who saw drug abuse because the nation's "number one problem" was simply 2-6%. The figure grew through the remainder of the 1980s till, in September 1989, it reached a noteworthy 64% – one of the foremost intense fixations by the American public on any issue in polling history. However, the figure plummeted to less than 10%, as the media lost interest. The draconian policies enacted throughout the hysteria remained, however, and continued to result in escalating levels of arrests and incarceration.

Although Bill Clinton advocated for treatment instead of incarceration throughout his 1992 presidential campaign, after his initial few months in the White House he reverted to the warfare strategies of his Republican predecessors by continuing to escalate the drug war. Notoriously, Clinton rejected a U.S. Sentencing Commission recommendation to eliminate the inequality between crack and powder cocaine sentences. He also rejected, with the encouragement of drug czar General Barry McCaffrey, Health Secretary adult female Shalala's recommendation to finish the federal ban on funding for syringe access programs. Yet, a month before leaving office, Clinton declared in a Rolling Stone interview that "we extremely need a reexamination of our entire policy on imprisonment" of individuals United Nations agency use drugs, and said that marijuana use "should be decriminalized."

At the height of the drug war hysteria in the late 1980s and early Nineties, a movement emerged seeking a new approach to drug policy. In 1987, Arnold Trebach and Kevin Zeese supported the Drug Policy Foundation – describing it as the "loyal opposition to the war on drugs." Prominent conservatives such as William Buckley and Milton Friedman had long advocated for ending drug prohibition, as had civil libertarians such as old ACLU govt Director Ira Glasser. In the late Eighties, they were joined by Baltimore civil authority Kurt Schmoke, Federal decide Robert Sweet, Princeton academician Ethan Nadelmann, and other activists, scholars and policymakers.

In 1994, Nadelmann founded The Lindesmith Center because of the first U.S. project of George Soros' Open Society Institute. In 2000, the growing Center merged with the Drug Policy Foundation to create the Drug Policy Alliance.

THE NEW MILLENNIUM: NEW SENSIBLE DRUG POLICY

George W. Bush arrived in the White House as the drug war was running out of steam – nonetheless he allocated a lot of money than ever to it. His drug czar, John Walters, zealously focused on marijuana and launched a major campaign to promote student drug testing. whereas rates of illicit drug use remained constant, overdose fatalities rose rapidly.

The era of George W. Bush also witnessed the rapid step-up of the militarization of domestic drug law enforcement. By the end of Bush's term, there have been about 40,000 paramilitary-style SWAT raids on Americans every year – principally for non-violent drug law offenses, often misdemeanors. While federal reform mostly stalled below Bush, state-level reforms finally began to slow the growth of the drug war.

Politicians now routinely admit to having used marijuana, and even cocaine, once they were younger. once Michael Bloomberg was questioned throughout his 2001 mayoral campaign about whether or not he had ever used marijuana, he said, "You bet I did – and I enjoyed it." Barack Obama also frankly discussed his previous cocaine and marijuana use: "When I was a kid, I indrawn frequently – that was the point."

Public opinion has shifted dramatically in favor of smart reforms that expand health-based approaches while reducing the role of criminalization in drug policy.

Marijuana reform has gained unprecedented momentum throughout the Americas. Alaska, California, Colorado, Nevada, Oregon, Maine, Massachusetts, Washington State, and Washington D.C. have legalized marijuana for adults. In Dec 2013, Uruguay became the first country in the world to lawfully regulate marijuana. In Canada, Prime Minister Justin Trudeau plans legitimate marijuana for adults by 2018.

In response to a worsening overdose epidemic, dozens of U.S. states passed laws to increase access to the drug antidote, naloxone, as well as "911 Good Samaritan" laws to encourage individuals to seek medical help within the event of associate degree drug.Yet the assault on American voters and others continues, with 700,000 people still arrested for marijuana offenses each year and virtually five hundred people still behind bars for nothing more than a drug law violation.

President Obama, despite supporting much successful policy changes – such as reducing the crack/powder sentencing inequality, ending the ban on federal funding for syringe access programs, and ending federal interference with state medical marijuana laws – did not shift the bulk of drug policy funding to a health-based approach.

Now, the new administration is threatening to require the country to thread backward toward an Eighties style warfare. President Trump is calling for a wall to keep drugs out of the country, and Attorney General Jeff Sessions has made it clear that he does not support the sovereignty of states to legalize marijuana, and believes "good people don't smoke marijuana."

Progress is inevitably slow, and even with an administration hostile to reform there is still unprecedented momentum behind drug policy reform in states and localities across the country. The Drug Policy Alliance and its allies will continue to advocate for health-based reforms like marijuana legitimation, drug lawmaking, safe consumption sites, naloxone access, bail reform, and more.

"Reefer Madness"

The widely popular film "Reefer Madness," which aired in 1936, fueled parental concern over marijuana use and unfolded the fear that, should American youths consume marijuana, it would invariably corrupt them and give rise to crime and sex.

Although, people eventually began to become more educated about the actual effects of cannabis use, the film and culture encompassing it permeated the society deeply and reflected marijuana as a drug of abuse compared to a lot of dangerous substances -- a stereotype that still exists today.Still, with the recent craze over marijuana stocks and corporations, some are claiming another kind of proverbial "reefer madness" is going on.

FIRST LEGALIZATION OF MEDICAL MARIJUANA

Through the Compassionate Use Act of 1996, California officially became the Delaware to legalize medical marijuana for use by patients with chronic illnesses.Following its footsteps, the Nineties saw the legitimation in four other states plus Washington D.C. for medical marijuana, including Oregon, Washington, Alaska, and Maine. By the early 2000s, more states -- now as well as Nevada, Montana, Rhode Island, Hawaii, Green Mountain State and Land of Enchantment -- passed medical marijuana laws.

Since 2010, sixteen states have legalized the medical use of marijuana.Washington state and Green Mountain State were the primary two states to vote to legalize the recreational use of marijuana in 2012. Colorado's Proposition sixty-four made adult possession (those over twenty-one years of age) and business sale legal.Several states followed, currently leaving recreational marijuana legal in nine states and Washington D.C.

STATES THAT HAVE LEGALIZED MARIJUANA (IN SOME WAY)

As of 2018, there are thirty states plus Washington D.C. that have legalized marijuana in some form. Those states include Alaska, Arkansas, Arizona, California, Colorado, Connecticut, Delaware, Washington D.C., Florida, Hawaii, Illinois, Louisiana, Maine, Maryland, Massachusetts, Michigan, Minnesota, Montana, New Hampshire, Nevada, New Jersey, New Mexico, New York, North Dakota, Ohio, Oregon, Pennsylvania, Rhode Island, Vermont, Washington and West Virginia.

CHAPTER 5

WHAT'S NEXT FOR CANNABIS?

The North American Cannabis market made an astounding $9.7 billion last year -- up thirty-third from the previous year. And, according to their estimates, the legal marijuana industry is projected to generate $32 billion of overall international economic impact by 2022. Additionally, one in four young adults uses marijuana, according to a Gallup poll in 2018. And, with sixty-fourth of Americans supporting the legalization of marijuana, it seems as if federal group action isn't too far off.

Corporations and industries alike seem to be revving up for the inevitable widespread group action. In fact, Coca-Cola recently announced intentions to force an entry into the cannabis industry with an infused drink. And whereas Aurora Cannabis opposition. (ACBFF) may not be their supposed partner, it is clear that the alcohol business is trying to capitalize on the enormous emerging market. Experts predict that 2019 is going to be a huge year for the marijuana industry.

In 2018, pot reached a tipping point. A transparent majority of Americans now need to see the drug made totally legal. California and North American country began selling marijuana to anyone over twenty-one. Company behemoths like Altria (parent company of Marlboro cigarettes) and Constellation

Brands (parent of Corona brew and Svedka vodka) made multi-billion greenback weed investments. And Senate Majority Leader Mitch McConnell (R-KY) managed to include hemp legalization in the 2018 Farm Bill — actual legalizing every part of the cannabis plant except for consciousness-altering drug.

But pot prohibition is not over. Well over 0.5 million people are still put behind bars for possession every year. Smoking weed or working for a pot company will still threaten your housing, employment, immigration standing, finances, and freedom. Cannabis business models, regulative environments and market valuations shift on a daily basis.

THE FATE OF CANNABIS IN 2019

What happens in 2019 will undoubtedly have an effect on each of those problems. To better understand wherever weed is headed in the next twelve months, here are experts' predictions for 2019:

First up, the good news. "Within the next two years, a majority of the United States will have adult-use legal cannabis," predicts an old bigwig in cannabis political fund-raising. "And some of that, roughly half of that, could happen through state legislatures." Although Vermont legalized the possession and use of cannabis through the legislature, all nine of the states that legalized adult-use sales and commercial production have done so via ballot initiative. However in 2019, politicians can finally catch up with their constituents. States that might potentially legalize through the general assembly embody New York, New Jersey, Connecticut, and Illinois.

Meanwhile, movements to get a group action initiative on the ballot in 2020 area unit is underway in states like Arizona and Ohio. All this could mean that Congress is finally about to take federal marijuana legalization seriously in 2019, right? Well, maybe. A Colorado-based cannabis lobbyist in the UN agency who has spent the past few years in Washington D.C. working on behalf of some of the country's biggest weed operators, is cautiously optimistic concerning the 2019 chances for the narrow and pragmatic bill, the STATES Act, that he helped put together. Co-sponsored by a fraction of senators, the STATES Act would provide anyone following state marijuana laws a reprieve from federal consequences — which means weed businesses could, at long last, get bank accounts, take tax deductions and stop freaking out about potential criminal liability.

As for the 2018 Farm Bill, it's not yet clear what the regulatory landscape will look like for CBD in 2019. Edgar Allen Poe believes researchers will soon be able to access CBD while not jumping through the hoops necessary to acquire a Schedule I drug license from the Drug Enforcement Agency, that could finally enable scientists to produce a lot of evidence of the compound's uses and dose. Still, several people in the cannabis business are concerned about what the exact pointers can look like on the commercial production side, and how the rollout will go.

For business owners who have been involved in the weed game for a while, another aspect of the 2018 Farm Bill has proven a disturbing sign of the times: anyone with a drug law-breaking conviction in the past ten years won't be allowed to participate in the legal hemp and CBD market.

Experts predict that there will be huge growth in the forms of cannabis products offered.

The drug-felony provision in the Farm Bill cuts to the heart of one in all the biggest unresolved problems facing the marijuana movement in 2019: the persistence of the illicit market and the struggle to accommodate folks who are illegally selling or growing marijuana for years. It is now wide acknowledged that blackball folks with drug law-breaking convictions from the cannabis industry is racist, as white folks with experience on the illicit marijuana market are far less likely to be arrested or convicted. however even without a criminal record, making the transition from outlaw to mogul has proven incredibly difficult, and lots of of the people in the UN agency who have tried have already given up.

"The reality is that the people that are in the illicit market have been there for decades," says an expert."Unless they cut back the barrier to entry and reduce the amount of greed and taxation, they're going to feed the illicit market, and the legal market is going to finish up failing."

"The last time we had a tendency of a funding boom like this was for HIV research in the Nineties," says one researcher.

Taxes, in particular, are a thorny issue. Local and state governments generally consider pot taxes to be a primary incentive for group action, however, if tax rates area unit too high, fewer growers and dispensaries will try to go legal. Already, lax oversight and an oversupply of legal cannabis in states like Washington have led to diversion rates of at least 30% — which means at a minimum a few third of legal pot is being sold on the illicit market. Meanwhile, in places like California, Canada, and Michigan, hundreds of illegal front marijuana dispensaries compete with legal vendors, consistently undercutting them on price. These illicit operators have stated over and over again that they cannot afford to survive in the highly taxed and regulated legal market.

In 2017 and 2018, places like Oakland and Sacramento garnered bootlicking headlines for setting the lofty goal of lawmaking solutions to the catastrophic and racially disproportionate impact of the War on Drugs. However moving into 2019, California cannabis operators of all colors and political stripes currently usually describe equity as a well-intended idea that is failing in practice. The words "tokenism" and "paternalistic" come up quite a number of times. .

Since nothing about marijuana policy ever makes any sense, U.S. cannabis companies that are directly involved in the plant cannot be listed on U.S. stock exchanges, however, some of those companies are listed on Canadian stock exchanges. And, since they're attracting such a lot of American investors, some major Canadian cannabis companies are now listed on several distinguished U.S. stock exchanges. These Canadian operators are the businesses taking on multi-billion dollar investments from the alcohol and tobacco industries. These are the companies that little businesses concern, resent, or hope will see them as an acquisition target. These are the companies that have already taken the path to European countries and Israel, laying the groundwork to dominate the global marijuana industry for years to come.

"On a global level for the industry, 2019 will be characterized by product innovation," says the corporate executive of a Canadian cannabis company.

"On a world level for the industry, 2019 can be characterized by product innovation," an expert says. "We have this influx of specialists and creative people from other industries — whether or not its food, beverage, tobacco, cosmetics — coming back into the space and working with cannabis experts on developing products."

Other CEOs and financial analysts echoed this prediction: a lot of outsiders can arrive with more money and more experience, and that they will reshape the cannabis industry to look a lot of like where they came from.

CHAPTER 6

THE DIFFERENT KINDS OF CANNABIS

There are three distinct types of marijuana leaves and they sit among three different categories; Sativa, Indica and Hybrid. The plants of Cannibis indica and Cannabis sativa have been around since the 18th century with Cannabis Hybrid as a new introduction. Hybrid indicates the mixing of seeds from different geographic locations around the world.

A much revered pastime in the cannabis culture is to perfect the growing and harvesting. The flavors and diversity is comparative to how many cookies exist around the world, it's endless. There are many a specialists too, choosing what they buy based on the strain alone. It should be mentioned that most of the marijuana offered is a mix of Sativa and Indica.

1. INDICA

The origin is believed to come from the Hindu "Kush" region close to Afghanistan. Anyone who knows anything about marijuana knows that Kush is really strong weed. In this area of Afghanistan, the strain developed thick coats of resin as a mean of protecting themselves due to the harsh climate. Characteristics of Indica include flowering time, yields, geography of where seeds came from and various flavors. Some of the epic names given to top flavors include; Purple Haze, Granddaddy Purple and Northern Lights.

The Indica strain is a more relaxing effect with the tendency of making you want to hang out on the couch. I sometimes wonder if the gaming companies are in cahoots with the marijuana industry as they seem to go hand in hand.

2. SATIVA

The Sativas strain alternatively has energizing effects which is why they're often used for morning or afternoon use. This strain of marijuana is used primarily for depression and exhaustion. Its morphology is a growth of up to 20 feet high, it is narrow with loose branches.

The effects of Sativa are said to be uplifting and allow you to bring your creative side out. Medicinally, it can treat ADD and mood disorders. Some of the more popular flavors under the Sativa strain include Sour Diesel, Jack Herer and Lemon Haze.

3. HYBRID

There are many variables for the two ancient strains which is where Hybrid comes in. The seeds of many geographical areas are cross germinated to balance marijuana with both strains. This offers the marijuana user a balance between the two so you get the best of both worlds.

MEDICAL MARIJUANA

For thousands of years, different cultures have been using marijuana for its medicinal properties. In the 1830s, Irish doctor Sir William Brooke O'Shaughnessy discovered marijuana's benefits in treating nausea and pain in cholera patients in India. This lead to the widespread sale and use of cannabis as a cure for a variety of stomach ailments in Europe and even the United States -- primarily by doctors and pharmacies in the later 19th century.

Today, different compounds of marijuana -- like CBD and THC -- are being used to treat a variety of conditions like epilepsy and cancer-related ailments.

CBD (CANNABIDIOL)

CBD is the non-psychoactive component of marijuana that is often associated with its health benefits, including relieving anxiety and depression, while THC, the psychoactive component, induces sleep or drowsiness. Because CBD and THC do not operate the same way (and have different effects on the body), they have seen varying uses over the years -- specifically in the medical arena.

The first CBD-based drug, Epidiolex, was approved earlier in 2018 by the FDA to treat epilepsy. Experts believe it may trigger wider FDA approval of CBD-based drugs and medications. The drug's approval can be seen as a snowball effect that could redirect patients from more dangerous alternatives.

THC

THC, or tetrahydrocannabinol, is the psychoactive component of marijuana that has more frequently been the source of controversy regarding the plant's usage. While traditional recreational use of the cannabis plant may have involved smoking high levels of THC for religious or other ceremonies, recent centuries have seen the compound transformed into anything from tinctures to gummies and edibles. In addition, synthetic THC has also been used to create the drug Marinol, used for treating nausea and vomiting associated with cancer treatment.

CANNABINOIDS AND WHERE THEY CAN BE FOUND

The word cannabinoids refers to every chemical substance, regardless of its origin or structure, that joins the cannabinoid receptors of the body and brain and that have similar effects to those produced by the plant Cannabis Sativa L. We know it is a large and varied group of substances that can be classified in several ways, but the most useful way to understand the cannabinoid diversity is the following:

PHYTOCAN-NABINOIDS

Phytocannabinoids make reference to the kinds of compounds characterised by 21 carbon atoms which only show in nature in the plant Cannabis Sativa L. Around 70 phytocannabinoids have already been found, including their acidic and neutral forms, their analogous and other transformation products. The plant is just able to synthesise the phytocannabinoids directly in their non-psychoactive forms. Therefore, the main phytocannabinoids present in fresh plant material are Δ9-THCA, CBDA, CBGA y CBCA. However, the carboxyl group is not very stable and it is easily lost as CO_2 under the influence of heat or light, which causes the transformation in the active neutral forms. The acidic phytocannabinoids suffer partial decarboxylation in the drying and curing process of buds; subsequently, acidic phytocannabinoids and some of their active neutral forms (Δ9-THC, CBD, CBG y CBC) are mainly found in the plant dry material. A large drying process of the plant material would generate the reduction of acidic phytocannabinoids and the increase of the neutral ones. When the plant is smoked or cooked every acidic cannabinoid suffers decarboxylation in its neutral form due to the influence of heat.

The method normally used in the decarboxylation of small quantities of Cannabis plant material (i.e. 20 grams) consists of placing it in an oven at 120 ºC for a minimum period of 20 minutes. Cooking the Cannabis in butter or oil will also initiate the process for as long as necessary. It is interesting that the most studied phytocannabinoid, Δ9-THC, in its neutral form is the main one responsible for the psychoactive effects caused by Cannabis intake, while it does not show psychoactive activity in its acidic form Δ9-THCA.

ENDOCAN-NABINOIDS

Endocannabinoids are produced by almost every organism in the animal kingdom. They are natural endogenous ligands produced by human and animal organisms that join the cannabinoid receptors. Both endocannabinoids and cannabinoid receptors form the endocannabinoid system, which is involved in a large variety of physiological processes, such as the control of the neurotransmitters release, the pain perception and the cardiovascular, gastrointestinal and liver functions. The two main endocannabinoids found are the anandamide (Narachidonoylethanolamine or ANA) and 2-arachidonoylglycerol (2-AG). Endocannabinoids are the molecules that act as natural key for the main cannabinoid receptors CB1 and CB2 and cause their activation and subsequent action. CB1 is mainly located in the central nervous system and it is responsible for the effects mediated by neuronal processes and psychoactive 'secondary' effects. CB2 is mainly located in the immune system and it is responsible for the immunomodulatory effects. CB2 receptors have been recently discovered in the central nervous system, the microglial cells and they seem to be in certain neurons as well. However, it remains a quite controversial and debated issue.

SYNTHETIC CANNABINOIDS

The main difference between phytocannabinoids, endocannabinoids and synthetic cannabinoids is that the latter are fully synthetic and created in the laboratory. An example of it would be dronabinol (Δ9-THC synthetic), which is the active compound of MARINOL®, a medicine that comes in capsules and has been consumed in the US since 1985 to prevent nausea, vomiting, loss of appetite and loss of weight. Another example would be nabilone, that is the active substance of CESAMET®, a medicine approved for the nausea and vomiting control caused by cancer chemotherapy. Both medicinal products have been approved for these purposes in the US, United Kingdom, Switzerland, Canada and Spain. More recently, some selective cannabinoids for CB1 receptor, such as JHW-018 y JHW-073, have been used as psychoactive ingredients in smart drugs marketed as imitations of Cannabis effects. One of the names used for these drugs is "Spice". There is not much information about the effects of synthetic cannabinoids in humans, although some of them have already shown to cause more distress and panic than phytocannabinoids. Synthetic cannabinoids have been designed as research tools for cannabinoid scientific studies, however, they have never shown to be reliable for human consumption in clinical testing. In theory, they should have never left the laboratory where they where designed and synthesised.

WHAT PART OF THE PLANT ARE PHYTOCANNABI NOIDS PRODUCED IN?

It has been largely accepted that phytocannabinoids are mainly or fully synthesised and stored in small structures called glandular trichomes. Trichomes are present in most of the aerial surfaces of the plant. These structures together with cannabinoids are also found in most of terpenes (monoterpenes and sesquiterpenes), which provide each species with a different aroma, depending on their number and combination. This is the reason why it can be said that trichomes are the most interesting part of Cannabis for pharmacognosy experts.

Cannabis researchers speak of two types of non-glandular trichome (simple unicellular trichomes and natural killer trichomes) that have not been associated with terpenoid biosynthesis. Three types of glandular trichome have been found in female Cannabis plants: bulbous trichome, capitate-sessile trichome and capitate-stalked trichome. It has been shown that male plants have a fourth type of glandular trichome, the glandular trichome of the anthers which only has been found in the anthers.

Even though trichomes can be found in any male and female plant, its highest phytocannabinoid concentration (speaking in % of dry plant material) can be found in female inflorescence's bracts reaching 20% and 25%. Phytocannabinoids are more abundant in capitate-stalked trichome. This kind of trichome appears during the flowering period and forms the thickest cover in pistilated flowers' bracts. A high concentration of capitate-stalked trichome can also be found in the small leaves that go with flowers. Phytocannabinoids are less abundant in plant foliage leaves and stems, while they are quite rare or non-existent in the roots. There are not qualitative dissimilitudes within phytocannabinoids between the different parts of the plant, but there are quantitative ones. The role of phytocannabinoids in plants is unclear. The most plausible hypothesis is that they offer defensive properties against biotic stress (insects, bacteria and fungi) and abiotic stress (drying and ultraviolet radiation) of the plant.

HOW ARE PHYTOCANNABI NOIDS PRODUCED IN THE PLANT?

Neither the pathway nor the location of phytocannabinoid biosynthesis are fully known, however, some authors suggest that they are synthesised in specialised disc cells that appear in glandular trichomes. They are subsequently accumulated in the adjacent secretory cavity and finally emitted as resins, or their synthases are directly secreted in the secretory cavity.

An important structural variation of phytocannabinoids is found in the lateral alkyl chain. In fact, the alky group in the most common phytocannabinoid, $\Delta 9$-tetrahidrocannabinol ($\Delta 9$-THC), is a pentyl, while it is a propyl in its counterpart $\Delta 9$-THCV, named using the suffix "varin" or "varol". Such variations are explained by the fact that the geranyl pyrophosphate can be combined with the olivetolic acid and/or the divarinic acid. This is the starting point in the phytocannabinoids' biosynthesis, which results in the formation of the intermediate phytocannabinoids' cannabigerolic acid (CBGA) and/or cannabigevarolic acid (CBGVA) respectively. The intermediate CBGA/CBGVA is subsequently processed by $\Delta 9$-THC synthase, which converts CBGA/CBGVA into $\Delta 9$-THCA/$\Delta 9$-THCVA. Both the proportion between the propyl and pentyl intermediate phytocannabinoids and the presence of Δ9-THC synthase, are genetically determined.

All plants express CBC synthase, which fights for the same intermediate CBGA/CBGVA as CBD synthase and/or Δ9-THC synthase. In 'normal' Cannabis plants CBC synthase is active mainly in the early stage, which causes the detection of a higher proportion of this precise phytocannabinoid during the vegetative stage, if compared with the reproductive stage.

The products resulting from the acidic phytocannabinoids degradation, such as CBNA (cannabinolic acid) and CBLA (cannabicyclolic acid) appear as artefacts and are derived from several factors, namely; ultraviolet light, oxidation and isomerisation.

BASIC INTRODUCTION TO THE MAIN NON-PSYCHOACTIVE PHYTOCANNABINOIDS

The Cannabis plant contains many phytocannabinoids with weak or null psychoactivity, which, from a therapeutic point of view, could be much more promising than Δ9-THC.

CBD is an important non-psychotropic phytocannabinoid that produces a large amount of pharmacological, anti-oxidant and anti-inflammatory effects, among others, transmitted by several mechanisms. It has been clinically proven in cases of anxiety, psychosis and movement disorders, as well as to alleviate neuropathic pain in individuals suffering from multiple sclerosis.

CBDA does not join CB1 and CB2 cannabinoid receptors, although it is an inhibitor of selective COX-2 with anti-inflammatory effects. However, it can join certain vanilloids receptors, but its effects are not fully understood yet. In addition to this, it does act against proliferation.

CBG acts against proliferation and as an antibacterial. It is a ligand from CB2 cannabinoid receptor and an inhibitor of the re-absorption of anandamide. Furthermore, it is a vanilloids ligand.

CBC can cause hypothermia, sedation and hypoactivity in mice. It also acts as an anti-inflammatory, an antimicrobial and a soft analgesic. Moreover, it is a powerful antagonist of vanilloids and a weak inhibitor of the re-absorption of anandamide.

CHAPTER 7

WHAT IS CBD (CANNABIDIOL)

People take or apply cannabidiol to treat a variety of symptoms, but its use is controversial. There is some confusion about what it is and how it affects the human body. Cannabidiol (CBD) may have some health benefits, and it may also pose risks. Products containing the compound are now legal in many American states where marijuana is not.

Cannabidiol (CBD) is a naturally occurring compound found in the resinous flower of cannabis, a plant with a rich history as a medicine going back thousands of years. Today the therapeutic properties of CBD are being tested and confirmed by scientists and doctors around the world. A safe, non-addictive substance, CBD is one of more than a hundred "phytocannabinoids," which are unique to cannabis and endow the plant with its robust therapeutic profile.

CBD is closely related to another important medicinally active phytocannabinoid: tetrahydrocannabinol (THC), the compound that causes the high that cannabis is famous for. These are the two components of cannabis that have been most studied by scientists.

Both CBD and THC have significant therapeutic attributes. But unlike THC, CBD does not make a person feel "stoned" or intoxicated. That's because CBD and THC act in different ways on different receptors in the brain and body.

CBD can actually lessen or neutralize the psychoactive effects of THC, depending on how much of each compound is consumed. Many people want the health benefits of cannabis without the high – or with less of a high.

The fact that CBD is therapeutically potent as well as non-intoxicating, and easy to take as a CBD oil, makes it an appealing treatment option for those who are cautious about trying cannabis for the first time.

Many people are seeking alternatives to pharmaceuticals with harsh side effects – medicine more in synch with natural processes. By tapping into how we function biologically on a deep level, CBD can provide relief for chronic pain, anxiety, inflammation, depression and many other conditions.

Extensive scientific research – much of it sponsored by the U.S. government – and mounting anecdotal accounts from patients and physicians highlight CBD's potential as a treatment for a wide range of maladies, including (but not limited to):

- Autoimmune diseases (inflammation, rheumatoid arthritis)
- Neurological conditions (Alzheimer's, dementia, Parkinson's, multiple sclerosis, epilepsy, Huntington's chorea, stroke, traumatic brain injury)
- Metabolic syndrome (diabetes, obesity)
- Neuropsychiatric illness (autism, ADHD, PTSD, alcoholism)
- Gut disorders (colitis, Crohn's)
- Cardiovascular dysfunction (atherosclerosis, arrhythmia)
- Skin disease (acne, dermatitis, psoriasis)

CBD has proven neuroprotective effects and its anti-cancer properties are being investigated at several academic research centers in the United States and elsewhere. A 2010 brain cancer study by California scientists found that CBD "enhances the inhibitory effects of THC on human glioblastoma cell proliferation and survival." This means that CBD makes THC even more potent as an anticancer substance. Also in 2010, German researchers reported that CBD stimulates neurogenesis, the growth of new brain cells, in adult mammals.

HOW CBD WORKS

CBD and THC interact with our bodies in a variety of ways. One of the main ways they impact us is by mimicking and augmenting the effects of the compounds in our bodies called "endogenous cannabinoids" - so named because of their similarity to the compounds found in the cannabis plant. These "endocannabinoids" are part of a regulatory system called the "endocannabinoid system".

The discovery of the endocannabinoid system has significantly advanced our understanding of health and disease. It has major implications for nearly every area of medical science and helps to explain how and why CBD and THC are such versatile compounds – and why cannabis is such a widely consumed mood-altering plant, despite its illegal status.

The endocannabinoid system plays a crucial role in regulating a broad range of physiological processes that affect our everyday experience – our mood, our energy level, our intestinal fortitude, immune activity, blood pressure, bone density, glucose metabolism, how we experience pain, stress, hunger, and more.

All cannabinoids, including CBD, produce effects in the body by attaching to certain receptors. The human body produces certain cannabinoids on its own. It also has two receptors for cannabinoids, called the CB1 receptors and CB2 receptors.

CB1 receptors are present throughout the body, but many are in the brain. The CB1 receptors in the brain deal with coordination and movement, pain, emotions, and mood, thinking, appetite, and memories, and other functions. THC attaches to these receptors.

CB2 receptors are more common in the immune system. They affect inflammation and pain. Researchers once believed that CBD attached to these CB2 receptors, but it now appears that CBD does not attach directly to either receptor. Instead, it seems to direct the body to use more of its own cannabinoids.

CBD HEALTH BENEFITS

CBD may benefit a person's health in a variety of ways.

NATURAL PAIN RELIEF AND ANTI-INFLAMMATORY PROPERTIES

People tend to use prescription or over-the-counter drugs to relieve stiffness and pain, including chronic pain. Some people believe that CBD offers a more natural alternative.

Authors of a study published in the Journal of Experimental Medicine found that CBD significantly reduced chronic inflammation and pain in some mice and rats. The researchers suggested that the non-psychoactive compounds in marijuana, such as CBD, could provide a new treatment for chronic pain.

QUITTING SMOKING AND DRUG WITHDRAWALS

Some promising evidence suggests that CBD use may help people to quit smoking. A study found that smokers who used inhalers containing CBD smoked fewer cigarettes than usual and had no further cravings for nicotine.

A similar review, published in Neurotherapeutics found that CBD may be a promising treatment for people with opioid addiction disorders.The researchers noted that CBD reduced some symptoms associated with substance use disorders. These included anxiety, mood-related symptoms, pain, and insomnia.

More research is necessary, but these findings suggest that CBD may help to prevent or reduce withdrawal symptoms.

EPILEPSY

After researching the safety and effectiveness of CBD oil for treating epilepsy, the FDA approved the use of CBD (Epidiolex) as a therapy for two rare conditions characterized by epileptic seizures in 2018.

In the U.S., a doctor can prescribe Epidiolex to treat:

- Lennox-Gastaut syndrome (LGS), a condition that appears between the ages of 3 and 5 years and involves different kinds of seizures
- Dravet syndrome (DS), a rare genetic condition that appears in the first year of life and involves frequent, fever-related seizures

The types of seizures that characterize LGS or DS are difficult to control with other types of medication. The FDA specified that doctors could not prescribe Epidiolex for children younger than 2 years. A physician or pharmacist will determine the right dosage based on body weight.

OTHER NEUROLOGICAL SYMPTOMS AND DISORDERS

Researchers are studying the effects of CBD on various neuro-psychiatric disorders. Authors of a 2014 review noted that CBD has anti-seizure properties and a low risk of side effects for people with epilepsy.

Findings suggested that CBD may also treat many complications linked to epilepsy, such as neurodegeneration, neuronal injury, and psychiatric diseases.

Another study found that CBD may produce effects similar to those of certain antipsychotic drugs, and that the compound may provide a safe and effective treatment for people with schizophrenia. However, further research is necessary.

FIGHTING CANCER

Some researchers have found that CBD may prove to combat cancer. Authors of a review published in the British Journal of Clinical Pharmacology found evidence that CBD significantly helped to prevent the spread of cancer. The researchers also noted that the compound tends to suppress the growth of cancer cells and promote their destruction. They pointed out that CBD has low levels of toxicity. They called for further research into its potential as an accompaniment to standard cancer treatments.

ANXIETY DISORDERS

Doctors often advise people with chronic anxiety to avoid cannabis, as THC can trigger or amplify feelings of anxiousness and paranoia. However, authors of a review from Neurotherapeutics found that CBD may help to reduce anxiety in people with certain related disorders.

The authors noted that current treatments for these disorders can lead to additional symptoms and side effects, which can cause some people to stop taking them. No further definitive evidence currently links CBD to adverse effects, and the authors called for further studies of the compound as a treatment for anxiety.

TYPE 1 DIABETES

Type 1 diabetes results from inflammation that occurs when the immune system attacks cells in the pancreas. Research published in 2016 by Clinical Hemorheology and Microcirculation found that CBD may ease this inflammation in the pancreas. This may be the first step in finding a CBD-based treatment for type 1 diabetes.

A paper presented in the same year in Lisbon, Portugal, suggested that CBD may reduce inflammation and protect against or delay the development of type 1 diabetes.

ACNE

Acne treatment is another promising use for CBD. The condition is caused, in part, by inflammation and overworked sebaceous glands in the body.

A 2014 study published by the Journal of Clinical Investigation found that CBD helps to lower the production of sebum that leads to acne, partly because of its anti-inflammatory effect on the body. Sebum is an oily substance, and overproduction can cause acne.

CBD could become a future treatment for acne vulgaris, the most common form of acne.

ALZHEIMER'S DISEASE

Initial research published in the Journal of Alzheimer's Disease found that CBD was able to prevent the development of social recognition deficit in participants. This means that CBD could help people in the early stages of Alzheimer's to keep the ability to recognize the faces of people that they know.

This is the first evidence that CBD may slow the progression of Alzheimer's disease.

SIDE EFFECTS OF USING CBD

There is often a lack of evidence regarding the safety of new or alternative treatment options. Usually, researchers have not performed the full array of tests. Anyone who is considering using CBD should talk to a qualified healthcare practitioner beforehand.

The FDA have only approved CBD for the treatment of two rare and severe forms of epilepsy and when drugs do not have FDA approval, it can be difficult to know whether a product contains a safe or effective level of CBD. Unapproved products may not have the properties or contents stated on the packaging.

It is important to note that researchers have linked cannabis use during pregnancy to impairments in the fetal development of neurons. Regular use among teens is associated with issues concerning memory, behavior, and intelligence.

Although,CBD is generally well tolerated. Some people report that it makes them sleepy or drops blood pressure. Since there are cannabinoid receptors in the skin, you might notice dry skin after using CBD. But a thorough review showed that CBD DOES NOT affect:

- Sensory perception
- Alertness, awareness
- Consciousness

- Behavior
- Inhibitions
- Food intake
- Heart rate
- Blood pressure

The review found that extremely high chronic daily doses affected the liver metabolism and some fertility measures, but you need a lot of CBD to get there.

Just like grain and vegetable farmers, cannabis producers spray their plants with pesticides and synthetic fertilizers. So, you can end up with adverse effects from the chemicals that have nothing to do with the active ingredient, CBD. Research the brand and choose pure products without chemicals.

SIDE EFFECTS OF EPIDIOLEX

Concerning the product that the FDA approved to treat two types of epilepsy, researchers noticed following adverse effects in clinical trials:

- Liver problems
- Symptoms related to the central nervous system, such as irritability and lethargy
- Reduced appetite
- Gastrointestinal problems
- Infections
- Rashes and other sensitivity reactions
- Reduced urination
- Breathing problems

The patient information leaflet notes that there is a risk of worsening depression or suicidal thoughts. It is important to monitor anyone who is using this drug for signs of mood change. Research suggests that a person taking the product is unlikely to form a dependency.

HOW TO TAKE CBD

So you've decided to join the growing revolution of people using cannabidiol (CBD) for relief and support with anxiety, arthritis, pain, menopause symptoms, insomnia and other health issues. Now comes the truly hard decision: tinctures, topicals, vaporizers, edibles... Which is best for you? And how much should you take?

If you're overwhelmed by the wide variety of CBD products, you are not alone. Each method delivers CBD to your body in a different way, which affects what it can be used for and how often you'll want to take it. Adding to that confusion is the fact that each of our bodies responds differently to CBD, meaning there is no one-size-fits-all recommendation. That's why I have put together a guide to help you design a cannabinoid treatment plan that fits your individual health goals — whether you're choosing your first CBD product, or just optimizing your current routine.

CLARIFY YOUR GOALS

With more than 65 different targets throughout your body, CBD has a staggering variety of therapeutic properties. Focusing on just one or two or those properties will help you find the best product and dosage quicker.

Ask yourself what you want CBD to improve. Do you want emotional support? Do you have a lot of arthritic pain? Are you just curious to see if life is somehow "better" with it? Many people benefit from tracking their progress. You could use a score to rate your symptoms or try journaling about your current experience. Creating a baseline record will help you judge the effectiveness of your CBD treatment.

WHERE DOES THE CBD NEED TO REACH?

In order for this little molecule to be effective, it must get to where it's needed. For most health goals, figuring out the location of CBD's target will be straightforward.

If your target is located anywhere close to your skin or a mucous membrane (ie vagina), you could first try a localized product like a topical or suppository. This delivers the highest concentration of CBD exactly where you want it. Otherwise, CBD needs to travel through your bloodstream to reach its target — whether that's to your brain, immune system, or other locations. Vaporizers and oral products are best for this purpose.

WHAT'S YOUR TIME FRAME?

How long CBD works in your body is a balance between how you ingest it and how quickly your body eliminates it. Some methods deliver a sharp, quick peak of CBD, while others offer a slow, steadier concentration.

If you're looking for immediate, short-term relief, then inhaled products like a vaporizer might be ideal. On the other hand, if you want to maintain steady levels of CBD throughout the day, then an oral product would be more appropriate.

EVERYBODY'S DIFFERENT: FINDING YOUR DOSE

How well each method works varies from person to person, and is influenced by many factors so dosing is a highly individual process. It's always recommended to start with a very low dose to make sure you don't react poorly to any of the product's ingredients. Try one or two drops of an oral formulation, or a tiny puff off a vaporizer. This will be well below the recommended serving size listed on the product.

Then, wait until after the CBD has peaked and is leaving your system before trying a slightly higher dose. Wait at least an hour for vaporizers, and 6+ hours for an oral formula. You can take more sooner, but any effects you feel will be the cumulative result of both doses.

ENHANCING ABSORPTION

Even if you know how much CBD is in each serving, that value only represents the maximum amount that could be entering your body — most of that CBD will never reach your bloodstream or its targets. But there are tricks that can help increase the amount of CBD your body absorbs.

Before increasing how much you vape, experiment with different inhalation techniques. If you're taking an oral formulation, try holding it under your tongue or swishing it around your mouth before swallowing.

WAYS TO TAKE CBD

- ❖ **Oral** - Swallowed
- ➢ **Types**: CBD oil, tinctures, edibles, capsules, powder

Pathway to targets: When CBD is ingested, it passes through the digestive tract, where it's absorbed into the bloodstream and travels throughout your body.

Time-frame: This is the slowest route for CBD to reach its targets, but also the longest period of time that it's active. Peak bloodstream levels are reported anywhere between 1-6 hours. Best for long-term supplementation.

Other considerations:

Food. Food affects your body's ability to absorb CBD, and more cannabinoids are absorbed on a full stomach. CBD is fat-soluble, and consuming with a healthy dose of fats can increase the amount of CBD that reaches your bloodstream 3-fold — which is why Foria Basics contains MCT coconut oil.

Pay attention to THC. Swallowed products are first metabolized by your liver before circulating through your body (first-pass metabolism). If your CBD product contains THC (i.e it's a "full-spectrum CBD"), it could be converted to 11-hydroxy-THC, which is a strong intoxicant. Many people find that CBD helps counterbalance the "high" associated with THC, but if you are sensitive to THC, look for CBD from a hemp source.

Prescription drug interactions. As mentioned earlier, CBD could interfere with the processing of certain drugs by cytochrome p450. Because cytochrome p450 is most concentrated in the liver, ingested CBD is more likely than inhaled CBD to cause drug interactions.

Time in your mouth. Everything above applies to CBD that is swallowed immediately. However, while it sits in your mouth, it can be absorbed directly into your bloodstream.

- ❖ **Oral - Sublingual or "Buccal"**
  - ➢ **Types: CBD oil, tinctures**

Pathway to targets: CBD can be absorbed directly into your bloodstream from capillary-rich areas underneath the tongue, along the gums and cheek. From here, it avoids first-pass metabolism and is sent throughout your body.

Time-frame: This route gets CBD into your bloodstream faster than swallowing. Under the tongue (sublingual) is generally quicker than against the cheek (buccal). However, because most of the CBD will eventually be swallowed, peak bloodstream levels range from 0.5 - 5 hours.

Other considerations:

Food. When evaluating an oral spray, researchers discovered that the total amount of absorbed CBD increases 5-fold if the person has recently eaten. Chewing helps increase blood flow to your mouth, which could help increase absorption.

Increase surface contact. It's often suggested to keep CBD oil in your mouth for 1.5 minutes or more before swallowing. During this time, increase absorption by vigorously swishing the oil around your mouth and even between your teeth — this increases the surface contact between the oil and your capillaries.

- ❖ **Inhalation**
  - ➢ **Types: Vape pens, dabs, high-CBD cannabis**

Pathway to targets: When CBD is inhaled, it passes to the lungs where it rapidly passes into the bloodstream. Inhalation avoids first-pass metabolism.

Time-frame: This is the quickest way to get CBD circulating through your system, but it also is effective for the shortest period of time. Peak bloodstream levels are within 10 minutes.

Other considerations:

Inhalation technique. Based on studies with THC, inhalation can get anywhere from 2-56% of this molecule into your bloodstream based on your inhalation technique. Try this: use the vaporizer for the first half of your inhalation, then finish your inhalation with a deep breath of fresh air — get those molecules deep in there! (This technique will also minimize irritation if the vapor is a bit too hot, by mixing in cooler air.) On exhale, any vapor that you can see is lost, so instead of exhaling fully, start a partial exhale until you see vapor — then inhale all the way back in and repeat a few times until you see less vapor on the exhale.

Vapor Pen Hardware. Avoid cheap, disposable vape pens, and watch out for any that list "propylene glycol" in the ingredients. Look for higher-quality vape pens with ceramic heating elements, for a cleaner vapor.

- ❖ **Topical**
  - ➢ **Types: Creams, lotions**

Pathway to targets: Topical CBD diffuses across your skin and reaches local targets, like muscles, inflammatory cells, and pain-perceiving nerves. Very little, if any, enters the bloodstream — unless it is designed for transdermal activity.

Time-frame: Varies, depending on the target.

Other considerations:

Often paired. Topicals are great for on-the-spot treatment and arousal. But for long-term health goals, people often get the best results when they pair topicals with oral or inhaled CBD products.

- ❖ **Vaginal & Anal**
- ➢ **Types: Suppositories, sprays, creams in applicators**

Pathway to targets: CBD applied to the mucosal tissue of the vagina and anus have the strongest effect locally at muscles, inflammatory cells, and pain-perceiving nerves — similar to the way topicals work. However, because these areas are rich in capillaries, some CBD could be absorbed into the bloodstream.

Time-frame: For local targets like sexual pleasure or menstrual cramps, Foria's suppository (THC/CBD) and vulva spray (CBD & Kava) are active within minutes (and possibly up to an hour) after application. Absorption into the bloodstream is highly variable and has only been studied rectally. Any molecules entering the bloodstream through the rectum should peak within 2-8 hours.

Other considerations:

Vaginal differences. Absorption across the vaginal wall will vary with your age, vaginal pH, and where you are on your menstrual cycle.

Anal placement. Whether or not rectal suppositories deliver CBD into the bloodstream is highly variable between individuals. If the suppository also contains THC in a general cannabinoid formula, placement of the suppository into the lower rectum (closer to the sphincter) can help avoid first-pass metabolism and the risk of a more "stoned" feeling.

CBD SOURCES & QUALITY

Once you find your optimal CBD method and dosage, be aware that it may change if you switch products. Some manufacturers are less trustworthy than others, so different CBD sources may have different effects.

Your CBD Source Matters More than You Think.Research is changing the way that we look at cannabis and cannabis-related compounds. What was once widely stigmatized has become respected as an effective health and beauty supplement. The widespread legalization of cannabidiol (CBD) oil has seen demand for it increase exponentially.

In other words, CBD oil has gone from a controversial but trendy concept to a legitimate player on store shelves across the country. Once upon a time, any cannabis product was associated with "getting high." In reality, CBD can work independently of the psychoactive components of the plant to alleviate pain, swelling, and even some symptoms of anxiety and psychological disorders. The human endocannabinoid system has an impact on nearly every part of the body, modulating many physiological systems—and CBD has been shown to have positive effects on several ailments from pain to epilepsy.

The issue with the rise of CBD lies in this: the accelerating popularity of CBD oil is pushing some companies to source their products from less-than-reputable manufacturers.. I believe it's important that anyone purchasing hemp products should understand the dangers of getting something substandard:

LOW-QUALITY CBD CONSTITUENTS

With the 2014 "Farm Bill," industrial hemp (also called cannabis sativa) has become a major cash crop across the country. People that don't have the knowledge or resources to properly cultivate the crop are trying to push out inferior products.

Low-quality products often contain inconsistent levels of THC, the psychoactive component of cannabis which is widely controlled. You could end up selling or producing something that isn't entirely legal if you don't take the time to properly source your CBD from a trusted operation. It could also contain chemical solvents and byproducts that can inadvertently poison consumers over a long period of use. In short, poorly vetting your CBD oil could get you arrested and make people sick, neither of which are good for business.

In addition to those consequences, some products may not contain enough CBD to have the desired effect. Imagine a customer expecting to find some relief with a CBD tincture or pain spray, only to find that it's about as effective as a placebo. This isn't fair to those who could truly benefit from CBD, but end up giving up on it because of a bad experience with an inferior product. Knowledge is key when it comes to sourcing the highest-quality CBD.

THE ETHICAL MOTIVES OF CBD PRODUCTION

Not only is the CBD oil often polluted with chemical solvents, it's also being made in a way that puts workers at risk. The Occupational Safety and Health Administration (OSHA) has made an effort to improve working conditions, and many reputable operations are developing safety management systems in response. As the industry flourishes, state and federal organizations are expected to begin enforcing safety regulations on a much larger scale.

What does this mean for the production of CBD? Although the thought of regular OSHA inspections may not inspire joy in producers, it does mean that the quality of CBD oil will only improve from here. New safety standards as well as quality standards will help to set the high-end operations apart, allowing retailers to choose from a better pool of CBD distributors.

It also means a more ethical approach to the manufacturing process, which is incredibly important to companies that only want the best for customers and employees.

CHOOSING A CBD SUPPLIER

There are some fantastic sources of CBD as a supplemental dietary product out there, it's just a matter of knowing what to look for. Fortunately, there are numerous suppliers that are working to improve quality control standards in every capacity. There are several things to consider before you buy, use, or sell any CBD product, including:

ASK ABOUT SOIL QUALITY AND CHEMICAL FERTILIZERS

When growing any crop, it's important to keep in mind that the contaminants in the soil can carry over into the plant. If a farmer is using harsh chemical fertilizers or pesticides, they can be absorbed into the hemp. Once they're in the hemp, they carry over into the CBD oil. This means that if a consumer uses a tincture or even a topical rub, those chemicals are making their way into their body.

Hemp is what's known as a "hyperaccumulator." This is a plant that rapidly absorbs anything that's in the soil. Not only are chemicals an issue, but heavy metals can also make their way into the plant when it's grown on low-quality land. Know where the hemp was grown, and what was used to keep it healthy. High-quality hemp starts with rich soil and natural pesticides and fertilizers. U.S.-grown hemp is held to higher standards by the department of agriculture, and this information should be readily available.

TAKE THE EXTRACTION METHODS INTO CONSIDERATION

Even the highest quality hemp can produce low-quality CBD oil when the wrong extraction methods are used. If you wouldn't be okay with ingesting propane or butane, then you certainly don't want it being used as a solvent to extract your CBD oil. These methods are cheap, but they pollute the finished product and lead to inconsistent amounts of CBD.

Ethanol extraction is still affordable, and essentially uses grain alcohol to purify the oil while keeping the cannabinoid levels fairly consistent. While this is a largely acceptable method, the top-shelf method is supercritical CO_2 extraction. This combines carbon dioxide with freezing temperatures in a high-pressure environment to extract an extremely pure form of CBD oil. This may translate into a higher cost for consumers, but many believe it also produces a more effective oil.

UNDERSTAND FULL-SPECTRUM AND ISOLATES

To be fully informed about what you're ingesting or using, you should know the difference between CBD isolate and full-spectrum CBD. Whole plant or full-spectrum means making the CBD oil from the entire hemp plant, versus making it from isolates, or only parts of the plant. A whole plant approach creates a more consistent product that's generally considered more effective. However, use discernment—the final use for the CBD will dictate whether the whole plant or isolates are more appropriate.

LOOK OUT FOR THIRD PARTY TESTING

Third party testing is a fail-safe. It checks that THC levels are within the acceptable range, the product is free of harmful chemicals, and that it has a consistent and therapeutic level of CBD. All of this is essential when choosing a CBD oil or product to fulfill a specific purpose. It also helps to establish the legality of the products before shipping them to a less "cannabis-friendly" state.

CBD: CAN YOU TAKE TOO MUCH?

If you're worried about taking too much, we recoommend speaking with a trusted medical professional before embarking on your CBD journey. Whether you're a first-time user or an experienced user, understanding how CBD works and how to use it can be somewhat confusing, especially since the industry is so new.

While there are tons of information about the benefits of CBD, there are few about properly dosing CBD. To make things more confusing, unlike with other supplements, The FDA has not created a Recommended Daily Intake (RDI) for CBD, which means CBD does not have an official serving size.

Because of this, consumers are blindly estimating their dosages based on recommendations from brands and companies they buy their CBD from. Or even worse... friends who are uncertified and claim to be "experts" simply because they use CBD.

"Take a drop of CBD per day," is one of the most common dosage recommendations we hear. While this can definitely be a dosage, there's no way to tell if its the right dosage for the given individual as it doesn't take into account important factors such as:

- The concentration of CBD
- The weight of the individual

- The individual's body chemistry
- The severity of the condition being treated

With that being said, there isn't a "one size fits all" dosage, and there will be some trial and error while gauging your proper dosage. Neuroscientists explain that, as our body's physiology changes, so do the receptors in our Endocannabinoid System (ECS), which are directly responsible for interactions with CBD. As a result, optimal CBD dosages will shift throughout an individual's lifetime.

In other words, there isn't necessarily a universal CBD dosage. So how much CBD should you take then? Use these 3 simple tips to find out:

HOW TO CHOOSE YOUR CBD DOSAGE

1. Estimate your dosage based on your body weight

As with most substances, individuals with more body mass will require more CBD to experience its effects. With that being said, a good rule of thumb to determine your proper CBD dosage is to take 1–6MG of CBD for every 10 pounds of body weight based on the individual's level of pain. For example, 20MG-33MG would be a great starting dosage for a 200 lb patient, while 15MG-25MG would be best for another who weighs 150 lb.

2. START SMALL AND INCREASE GRADUALLY

Let's say you have a friend who weighs no more than 150 pounds and takes 50MG of CBD twice per day, which he claims provides all kinds of benefits. Since you are approximately the same weight, they recommend the same dosage for you.

Here's why this isn't the best way to choose your dosage:

Not only are we all made differently, we each have our own unique history with the use of substances, medications, supplements, and other things we put in our body. Because of this, we all have different body chemistry, and this will affect how our body reacts to CBD. As R.R Noall over at Herb puts it, "what works for your friend, may not work for you."

With that being said, it is important to first determine your initial dosage based on your weight, gauge how your body reacted to that amount of CBD, then increase gradually while continuing to monitor your body's reactions till you find the perfect dosage that works for your situation.

3. CONSULT YOUR PHYSICIAN

When in doubt, consult your physician, especially if you have an existing medical condition. While there aren't a ton of doctors who have experience with CBD, most doctors should have a good idea on how your body will react to CBD and can provide you a professional CBD dosage for your situation. So, now that you know how much CBD you should take, there lies another important question: How do you accurately measure your CBD dosage? Think about it: How much CBD is there in a single puff off your vaporizer, how much CBD is in a drop from your CBD tincture?

Without understanding how to properly measure your dosage, knowing how much CBD you should take is pretty much pointless. Especially when it comes to all the different ways to consume CBD.

HOW TO MEASURE YOUR CBD TINCTURE DOSAGE

Using a CBD tincture is one of the easiest ways to consume CBD. Simply fill the dropper, administer the oil under your tongue, then hold it there for 30 to 90 seconds before swallowing. But, how many drops of CBD oil should you take?

With some simple mathematics, that can be figured out. Being that the dropper is the tool being used to administer a CBD tincture, it is paramount to know how much CBD is in a single dropper. Once this is known, gauging how much CBD to be taken should be as easy as a quiet stroll in the park.

So how do you figure out how much CBD is in a dropper? Typically a dropper holds 1 ML of liquid. It is important to know how many milliliters are in a CBD tincture, that way, this simple formula can be used to determine how much CBD is in its dropper:

[Total CBD in Bottle] ÷ [Number of Milliliters in Bottle] = MGs of CBD in a Dropper

For example; there is a 30ml CBD tincture that has 1500MG of CBD:

1500 ÷ 30 = 50MG of CBD per dropper

Now, if a proper dosage of CBD is 25MG, and a single dropper of that 1500MG tincture contains 50MG, the dropper will be filled halfway. Of course, this method isn't 100% accurate, but it is more accurate than not measuring at all. Remember, start with a small dosage and gradually increase until you find your perfect dosage.

HOW TO MEASURE YOUR CBD VAPE DOSAGE

Vaping CBD can be done using a CBD e-liquid or CBD cartridge system. Both methods are fairly easy and offer an enjoyable experience. When using an e-liquid to vape CBD, you'd start by estimating how much CBD is in a dropper (just like with a tincture). Once you know this, you know how much CBD you are putting into a single tank. As you vape throughout the day, keep an eye on when you need to refill your tank, and how many times you need to refill your tank.

If your proper dosage of CBD is 25MG, and you are using a 1000MG bottle of CBD e-liquid, a single tank would contain approximately 33.33MG of CBD. That being said, to properly administer your dosage, you would vape a single tank periodically throughout the day. Again, not 100% accurate; but with regular monitoring, you will be able to quickly gauge your CBD intake.

THE BEST WAY TO DOSE CBD

Since the methods mentioned so far have only been semi-accurate, you're probably wondering: "So is there a 100% accurate way to take CBD?"

There certainly is. CBD Capsules. Because CBD capsules are filled with an exact amount of CBD, they provide a truly accurate way to dose CBD. If your optimal CBD dosage is 16MG-25MG, then simply buy a bottle of 20MG or 25MG capsules and you're good to go. Other consumption methods that are just as accurate include CBD applicators, CBD edibles, CBD Gummies, and CBD beverages; although they may not be as convenient as capsules.

CBD EXTRACTION METHODS

The purpose of CBD extraction is quite simple; to create the cannabinoid (and others) in a highly concentrated form to make it suitable for human consumption. You must use a plant material rich in CBD such as special cannabis strains or hemp.

Special Strains such as AC/DC and Charlotte's Web have a high CBD concentration (up to 18% in some cases) and a low THC concentration (as little as 5%). You need a favorable CBD/THC ratio because even in cases where plants have a THC concentration of up to 6%, the extra high CBD content should hopefully render the psychoactive effects of THC inert.

Various strains of industrial hemp are another way to extract CBD. They are grown around the world legally; including in India, China and several countries in Western Europe. One of the most popular industrial hemp strains is Fedora 17 because it has an extremely low THC content which means that any CBD extracted from it has virtually no psychoactive effects. CBD oil made from hemp is legal in almost every country around the world including in all 50 states in the U.S. because of the negligible THC content.

Without further ado, let's look at the 4 most common CBD oil extraction methods:

1 – THE CO2 CANNABIS EXTRACTION METHOD

This form of CBD extraction is actually divided into supercritical, subcritical and 'mid-critical' categories but supercritical is by far the most commonly used. In fact, it is the most regularly used extraction method of all because it is safe and provides a pure end product.

In simple terms, CO_2 cannabis extraction uses pressurized carbon dioxide (CO_2) to pull CBD (and other phytochemicals) from the plant. CO_2 acts like a solvent at certain temperatures and pressures but possesses none of the dangers. While it is safe and effective, it also involves extremely expensive equipment. The rather sophisticated machines used for the purpose work to freeze the CO_2 gas and compress it into a supercritical cold liquid state.

CO_2 typically behaves like a gas at standard pressure and temperature, and is easily changed to a solid while in this state; the solid version of the gas is known as 'dry ice.' Using the aforementioned equipment in a lab, you can turn CO_2 gas into a liquid by ensuring the temperature drops below -69 degrees Fahrenheit while increasing the pressure to over 75 pounds per square inch (psi). At this stage, you have your starting point for CO2 Cannabis extraction.

Once you have the liquid CO2, the next step is to increase the temperature and pressure past the point where the liquid becomes 'supercritical.' This term means the CO2 is now capable of adopting properties halfway between a gas and liquid simultaneously. Effectively, the supercritical CO2 is capable of filling a container (like gas) while also maintaining density (like a liquid). When CO2 is in its supercritical state, it is ideal for chemical extraction because it won't cause the denaturing or damage that would make it unfit for human consumption.

Regarding extracting the CBD oil using this technique, you simply begin with liquid CO2 and raise its pressure via a compressor. You must also raise its temperature using a heater. The next step involves passing the supercritical carbon dioxide through some high-quality cannabis which should be in an extractor. Now, the CO2 will pull the essential trichomes and terpene oils out of the plant.

The solution gets passed via a separator and broken down into its requisite parts. The good stuff (including trichomes and terpene) is sent to the collection container. Meanwhile, the supercritical CO2 goes through a condenser and turned back into a liquid. Finally, the liquid goes to a special storage tank and can be used to begin the process all over again.

Subcritical

This form of extraction involves low temperature and low pressure. Subcritical extractions take longer than their supercritical counterpart and also produce a smaller yield. While it retains the terpenes, essential oils and other sensitive materials, it doesn't extract larger molecules such as chlorophyll, omega 3 & 6. Subcritical extraction is less likely to damage terpenes. Mid-critical is simply a general range between subcritical and supercritical. Some companies combine super-critical and subcritical to create a full-spectrum CO2 cannabis extract. They use the subcritical extraction method to separate the drawn out oil and draw out the very same plant material using supercritical pressure. The oils are then homogenized into one which creates a unanimated oil. This is known as the CO2 Total Extraction Process.

PROS OF CO2 CANNABIS EXTRACTION

- Safety: CO_2 is a common food additive and is used to produce carbonated soft drinks for example.
- Effectiveness: CO_2 has been used as an extraction solvent for years by food companies. It is used to remove caffeine from coffee and as an extraction solvent when producing essential oils.
- Purity: The cannabinoids produced are potent and free of chlorophyll with minimal risk of contaminants.

CONS OF CO2 CANNABIS EXTRACTION

- Expensive: You can only complete the process with the aid of extremely expensive equipment; estimates suggest the kit costs around $39,000.
- Technical Ability: CO2 Cannabis extraction is not something that should be attempted by an amateur chemist.

2 – THE OLIVE OIL EXTRACTION METHOD

While other liquids such as ethanol can be used in this process, olive oil is the most commonly used substance for this extraction which can be performed at home. The first step involves ensuring the raw plant material is decarboxylated. In layman's terms, it means you have to heat the plant at a certain temperature for a specific length of time to activate the plant's chemicals.

Most experts recommend heating at 248 degrees Fahrenheit for 60 minutes or at 284 degrees Fahrenheit for 30 minutes. Once this step is completed, add the plant material to the olive oil and heat to 212 degrees Fahrenheit for up to 2 hours (and at least 1 hour). This process should result in the extraction of the cannabinoids, and ultimately, you should receive oil with the CBD content you require.

PROS OF THE OLIVE OIL EXTRACTION METHOD

- Very Safe: You won't blow yourself up using this method to get CBD!
- Inexpensive: You can set everything up at home without breaking the bank.

CONS OF THE OLIVE OIL EXTRACTION METHOD

- Perishable: Regardless of whether your cannabis in-fused oil is high in CBD or THC, it is highly perishable so you must store it in a cool, dark place as soon as possible.
- Low Yields: This form of extraction only produces fairly low yields, so there is no possibility of a company using it due to the labor intensive nature of the method.

3 – THE DRY ICE EXTRACTION METHOD

The dry ice extraction method is another method of CBD extraction that can be performed at home although it takes a bit more time and effort than its olive oil equivalent. As well as the cannabis plant itself, you'll need the following equipment:

- Around 3 pounds of dry ice.
- A large piece of Plexiglas or a mirror.
- A paint scraper or putty knife.
- Thick gloves that are heat resistant and eye protection.
- A clean 5-gallon plastic bucket.
- 3 bubble hash mesh bags; sizes are 73, 160 and 220 microns.
- 3 large, clean glass jars for storage.

Put on your gloves and eye protection, chop up the cannabis plant into small pieces and place it in the bucket. Cover the plant with the dry ice and leave it for 3 minutes; it is best only to fill the bucket halfway; this process causes the freezing of the trichome resins. Fit the 73-micron bag over the bucket and sake the ice & plant combo for around 4 minutes; this knocks the frozen trichomes off.

Turn the bucket upside down on the Plexiglas and shake as much resin through the mesh bag as possible. Scrap the hash off the Plexiglas with your scraper and place it into one of the jars. Repeat with the 160 and 220-micron mesh bags, and you'll be rewarded with three different strains of extract.

PROS OF THE DRY ICE EXTRACTION METHOD

- Ease of Use: The steps above are very easy to follow.
- Clean: Unlike other methods, there is very little mess with dry ice extraction.
- Decent Yield: You'll end up with a lot more than if you use oil extraction.
-

CONS OF THE DRY ICE EXTRACTION METHOD

- Low-Quality: This is entirely dependent on the user, but you will ruin the quality of the product if you shake it for too long.
- Not Always Easy Getting Dry Ice: Depending on where you live, it isn't always so easy to get your hands on 3 pounds of dry ice unless you order it online.

4 – THE SOLVENT EXTRACTION METHOD

Ethanol, low-grade alcohol, and butane are among the most common substances used in Solvent Extraction. Although ethanol extracts the full range of cannabinoids and terpenes from the plant which makes the end product safe for consumption, it also extracts chlorophyll which may lead to some unpleasant side effects. You can remove the chlorophyll by filtering the extract, but you significantly reduce the oil's potency. Butane offers a stronger oil than ethanol, but it is more likely to contain solvents which could irritate the lungs.

All you have to do is add the liquid (whether it is butane, alcohol or ethanol) to the plant material. The extraction liquid will strip away the cannabinoids and flavor from the plant material but will probably take some of the green colorings too. Once you believe you have enough cannabinoids in liquid form, heat the liquid to evaporate it down to the CBD base oil.

PROS OF THE SOLVENT EXTRACTION METHOD

- Appropriate For Some Products: If you use high-grade alcohol, you may produce good quality oil suitable for vaping cartridges.
- Straightforward Process: Once you have the equipment, it isn't difficult to complete the process.

CONS OF THE SOLVENT EXTRACTION METHOD

- Extremely Dangerous: Butane and Ethanol are flammable, so it isn't worth starting a fire in your home to extract CBD in this manner.
- Potentially Harmful: As well as destroying plant waxes, this form of extraction may produce oil that contains chlorophyll or other harmful contaminants.

FINAL WORDS ABOUT CBD EXTRACTION

It is extremely important to understand the various CBD extraction methods as they have a major impact on the quality of the end product; not to mention your health. We don't recommend utilizing the solvent method because not only is it dangerous to make, it is also more likely to cause health problems. The cost of CO_2 supercritical extraction means it is not possible for 99.9% of readers although it is an excellent, safe and efficient method.

CHAPTER 8

REGULATORY STATUS OF CBD

On June 25, 2018, the U.S. Food and Drug Administration (FDA) announced its first-ever approval of a marijuana-derived pharmaceutical drug. Epidiolex (cannabidiol or CBD) was approved for the treatment of two rare, pediatric seizure disorders, Lennox-Gastaut syndrome and Dravet syndrome. On September 27, 2018, the Drug Enforcement Administration (DEA) announced its scheduling of Epidiolex - and future drug products containing CBD derived from marijuana with no more than 0.1 percent tetrahydrocannabinols - in Schedule V of the Controlled Substances Act (CSA). These events represent historical milestones in the journey of Cannabis from a source of textiles and medicines in the early nineteenth century to an illicit drug and now an FDA-approved drug.

Cannabidiol (CBD) is one of more than a hundred cannabinoids found in Cannabis sativa L. (Cannabis spp. or Cannabis), a plant more well-known colloquially as "marijuana" or hemp CBD was first isolated in 1940 and characterized structurally in 1963.[4,5] With projected retail sales of CBD products -hemp, marijuana and pharmaceutical - as high as $1.9 billion by 2020, CBD is poised to become the darling of the medical Cannabis movement.

THE COMPLEX LAWS SURROUNDING CBD

Despite its rapidly growing popularity and use, the regulatory status of CBD in the United States remains convoluted, even after the approval and scheduling of Epidiolex. The source of CBD is critically important in determining its legal status. The most common source, botanically speaking, is the plant Cannabis sativa L. (Cannabis), which encompasses both marijuana and hemp. There are various schema for differentiating marijuana from hemp (e.g. Genotype, phenotype, Drug-type Cannabis v. fiber-type Cannabis, etc.), but from a regulatory standpoint, the difference between marijuana and hemp is based on chemical composition, specifically as it relates to the concentration of delta-9 Tetrahydrocannabinol (THC), the primary intoxicating compound found in Cannabis. Hemp is legally defined as a cultivar of Cannabis sativa with low concentrations of THC. Although limitations on THC concentrations for hemp differ internationally, THC concentrations cannot exceed three tenths of one percent (0.3%) in the United States. Hemp-derived and marijuana-derived CBD each have their own unique regulatory status and consequent legal implications.

Despite the scheduling of Epidiolex, CBD from marijuana is still deemed a Schedule I controlled substance by the DEA pursuant to the 1970 Controlled Substances Act. As such, CBD from marijuana is deemed to have no accepted medical use, a lack of accepted safety for use under medical supervision, and a high potential for abuse.1,7-11 While the scheduling of Epidiolex represents the first time that the DEA has acknowledged that marijuana has a "currently accepted medical use", it did not change the regulatory status of CBD itself.

On May, 22, 2018, the DEA issued an internal directive which stated, "Products and materials that are made from the Cannabis plant and which fall outside the CSA definition of marijuana (such as sterilized seeds, oil or cake made from the seeds, and mature stalks) are not controlled under the CSA".12 Although these statements clarified that CBD derived from a source other than marijuana was not a controlled substance, they did not specifically state that CBD from industrial hemp was lawful. Furthermore, these parts of the plant are not viable sources of CBD. As a result, confusion remains.

CBD can also be extracted from some hemp cultivars. Historically, hemp has been bred as an industrial crop in order to produce fabrics, rope, and other textiles from its long stalks. Despite not being explicitly defined or mentioned in the CSA, has been considered a controlled substance by the DEA since the passage of the CSA in 1970.

On December 20, 2018, The Hemp Farming Act of 2018, S. 2667 (2018 Hemp Bill) became law and formally and definitively removed hemp from the list of controlled substances. The 2018 Hemp Bill redefines hemp as all parts of the Cannabis Sativa plant that do not exceed 0.3% delta-9 THC by dry weight, including "derivatives," "extracts" and "cannabinoids." Importantly, the 2018 Hemp Bill explicitly removes popular hemp products, including hemp-derived CBD, from the purview of the CSA.

Prior to the passage of the 2018 Hemp Bill, domestically cultivated hemp was only federally lawful when cultivated under a state-sanctioned pilot program. In 2017, a total of 23,343 acres of hemp were cultivated across 19 states. As of this writing, 41 states have passed legislation to allow them to take advantage of hemp pilot programs under the 2014 Farm Bill.15 Today, only a minority of the hemp-derived CBD products available in the US are derived from domestically cultivated hemp. This will change as the 2018 Hemp Bill fosters greater investment in this area.

In addition to industrial hemp, CBD may also be lawful if it is derived from "non-psychoactive hemp" imported into the US. Non-psychoactive hemp is the term used by the Ninth Circuit Court of Appeals in a pair of companion cases filed against the DEA by a national trade organization, the Hemp Industries Association (HIA), regarding a DEA rule, which would have made it illegal to import any hemp products that contained any THC, including trace amounts.16,17 In a February 6, 2004 ruling, the Court found that the DEA had exceeded its authority in enacting the rule and struck it down as void and unenforceable.

In its ruling – which did not specifically mention CBD – the Court used the term "non-psychoactive hemp", and in a footnote stated, "The non-psychoactive hemp used in Appellants' products is derived from industrial hemp plants grown in Canada and in Europe, the flowers of which contain only a trace amount of the THC contained in marijuana varieties grown for psychoactive use" (emphasis added). Confusion remains as to whether the Court, in effect, legalized the whole hemp plant for importation, including the "flowering tops", so long as it contains no more than trace amounts of THC, or whether it simply reiterated the mature stalks exception in a different context. That distinction has never been addressed. Cases addressing hemp, which both preceded and succeeded this ruling, do not resolve the issue.

Despite the confusion and the stance of the FDA and DEA, hemp-derived CBD products can currently be purchased both online and over-the-counter (OTC) throughout most of the country as if they were dietary supplements. In contrast, marijuana-derived CBD products can only be purchased by qualifying patients in states with medical marijuana laws or by consumers in states with adult-use/recreational laws.

BEFORE EPIDIOLEX

To complicate matters further, prior to the approval of Epidiolex, the FDA explicitly stated that "CBD products are excluded from the dietary supplement definition" because of CBD's status as an Investigational New Drug (IND) under the Food, Drug and Cosmetic Act (FD&C Act). CBD is no longer an Investigational New Drug (IND). It is an approved one. As a result, CBD cannot be included in a dietary supplement.

This preclusion is not entirely novel. In a somewhat similar case, Biostratum, a pharmaceutical company, requested the FDA take action against manufacturers of pyridoxamine-containing dietary supplements because Biostratum had submitted an IND application for pyridoxamine dihydrochloride. It took the FDA three and a half years to formally conclude that these products were in violation of its regulations. Products containing pyridoxamine and being sold as dietary supplements are not currently permitted.

There is another precedent which informs predictions of how the FDA might alter its enforcement approach going forward. In April 1997, Pharmanex, a dietary supplement manufacturer was advised by the FDA that its mevinolin-containing dietary supplement, named Cholestin, was a drug, not a dietary supplement. Mevinolin, also known as monocalin K, is a constituent of red yeast rice and has been shown to lower elevated cholesterol levels.Mevinolin is chemically identical to lovastatin (brand name Mevacor), an FDA-approved drug manufactured by Merck. The FDA concluded that Cholestin was manufactured to contain concentrations of lovastatin that exceeded traditional red yeast rice products, and the product was thus more similar to a drug than any red yeast rice product available OTC.23 While Cholestin is no longer available, many red yeast rice products remain on the market with naturally occurring concentrations of lovastatin.

In the Cholestin case, the FDA's argument hinged on the concentration of lovastatin in red yeast rice products exceeding some traditional standard. The vast majority of hemp-derived CBD oil products available today contain concentrations by weight of CBD below 5%, as compared to Epidiolex, which is ≥ 99% CBD. Given this precedent, it is possible, and perhaps even likely, that the FDA will restrict products that are enriched with isolated CBD but not hemp extracts that contain naturally occurring concentrations of CBD.

it is possible, and perhaps even likely, that the FDA will restrict products that are enriched with isolated CBD but not hemp extracts that contain naturally occurring concentrations of CBD.

With FDA-approval of Epidiolex, and the FDA's public proclamation that CBD products are excluded from the statutory definition of a dietary ingredient, the future of online and over-the-counter CBD products is uncertain. The FDA has the authority to enforce the Federal Food, Drug, and Cosmetic Act (FD&C Act) against products which are enriched with CBD. It is worth noting that the FDA is a public health agency with a myriad of competing priorities and a limited enforcement budget. When considering an enforcement action, the FDA weighs multiple factors, including benefits and harms.20 To date, harms associated with hemp-derived CBD products have been largely undocumented.

In the absence of strict FDA enforcement and oversight, widespread mislabeling of CBD products exists. Independent research has confirmed that the CBD content in almost 70% of CBD products available online could be mislabeled (43% of products were underlabeled and 26% were overlabeled for actual CBD content).The FDA sent warning letters to companies in 2015-16 for violations of FDA rule.The FDA has also sent cease and desist letters to companies for making drug claims about CBD products, including claims that they treat, or even cure cancer.

SO, IS CBD LEGAL?

Hemp-derived CBD isn't pot. It's not the same thing as THC and it's not psychoactive. Still, all cannabinoids are classified as Schedule I drugs in the US and Schedule II in Canada, due to a combination of politics, miscategorization, and a lack of understanding of the differences in chemical profiles and neuroscience.

Understandable — it's hard to get a tenacious politician with zero biology background to have a meaningful conversation about how the brain works.

You'll come across the claim that CBD is legal in all 50 states. Some retailers hold that CBD isn't the drug version of cannabis, and isn't subject to the same drug laws as medical marijuana is. You'll read that retailers are free to ship it anywhere they want to in the United States and in 40 additional countries. Since it's a dietary supplement, you can find it online, in health food stores, and at marijuana dispensaries.

CBD is a new supplement, and when something new comes onto the scene with some some amount of perceived crossover with something that's well-known and demonized, like marijuana, you end up with a big ol' gray area to contend with.

So, will you get busted? Depends on the state, depends on the employer, depends on the cop, depends, depends, depends. Most of the time, law enforcement has bigger fish to fry than the dude who's rubbing oil on his shoulder for bursitis, and still perfectly able to walk, talk, drive, and solve differential equations. But, there's always that one who wants to make a point.

CBD MISCONCEPTIONS

With the growing awareness of CBD as a potential health aid there's also been a proliferation of misconceptions. Find questions and responses to common misinformation.

It doesn't get you high, but it's causing quite a buzz among medical scientists and patients. The past year has seen a surge of interest in cannabidiol (CBD), a non-intoxicating cannabis compound with significant therapeutic properties. Numerous commercial start-ups and internet retailers have jumped on the CBD bandwagon, touting CBD derived from hemp as the next big thing, a miracle oil that can shrink tumors, quell seizures, and ease chronic pain—without making people feel "stoned." But along with a growing awareness of cannabidiol as a potential health aid there has been a proliferation of misconceptions about CBD.

> **CBD is medical. THC is recreational.** Oftentimes people say they are seeking "CBD, the medical part" of the plant, "not THC, the recreational part" that gets you high. Actually, THC, "The High Causer," has awesome therapeutic properties. Scientists at the Scripps Research Center in San Diego reported that THC inhibits an enzyme implicated in the formation of amyloid beta plaque, the hallmark of Alzheimer's-related dementia. The federal government recognizes single-molecule THC (Marinol) as

an anti-nausea compound and appetite booster, deeming it a Schedule III pharmaceutical, a category reserved for drugs with little abuse potential. But whole plant cannabis, which is the only natural source of THC, continues to be classified as a dangerous Schedule I drug with no medical value.

➢ **THC is the bad cannabinoid. CBD is the good cannabinoid.** The drug warrior's strategic retreat: Give ground on CBD while continuing to demonize THC. Diehard marijuana prohibitionists are exploiting the good news about CBD to further stigmatize high-THC cannabis, casting tetrahydrocannabinol as the bad cannabinoid, whereas CBD is framed as the good cannabinoid. Why? Because CBD doesn't make you feel high like THC does. This is quite another misconception to be rejected; reefer madness dichotomy in favor of whole plant cannabis therapeutics.

➢ **CBD is most effective without THC.** THC and CBD are the power couple of cannabis compounds—they work best together. Scientific studies have established that CBD and THC interact synergistically to enhance each other's therapeutic effects. British researchers have shown that CBD potentiates THC's anti-inflammatory properties in an animal model of colitis. Scientists at the California Pacific Medical Center in San Francisco determined that a combination of CBD and THC has a more potent anti-tumoral effect than either compound alone when tested on brain cancer and breast cancer cell lines. And extensive clinical research has demonstrated that CBD combined with THC is more beneficial for neuropathic pain than either compound as a single molecule.

➢ **Single-molecule pharmaceuticals are superior**

to 'crude' whole plant medicinals. According to the federal government, specific components of the marijuana plant (THC, CBD) have medical value, but the plant itself does not have medical value. Uncle Sam's single-molecule blinders reflect a cultural and political bias that privileges Big Pharma products. Single-molecule medicine is the predominant corporate way, the FDA-approved way, but it's not the only way, and it's not necessarily the optimal way to benefit from cannabis therapeutics. Cannabis contains several hundred compounds, including various flavonoids, aromatic terpenes, and many minor cannabinoids in addition to THC and CBD. Each of these compounds has specific healing attributes, but when combined they create what scientists refer to as a holistic "entourage effect" or "ensemble effect," so that the therapeutic impact of the whole plant is greater than the sum of its single-molecule parts. The Food and Drug Administration, however, isn't in the business of approving plants as medicine.

➤ CBD is not psychoactive. CBD is not an intoxicant, but it's misleading to describe CBD as non-psychoactive. When a clinically depressed patient takes a low dose of a CBD-rich sublingual spray or tincture and has a great day for the first time in a long time, it's apparent that CBD is a powerful mood-altering compound. Better to say, "CBD is not psychoactive like THC," than to simply assert that CBD is not psychoactive. CBD won't make a person feel stoned, but it can impact a person's psyche in positive ways.

➤ Psychoactivity is inherently an adverse side effect. According to politically correct drug war catechism, the marijuana high is an unwanted side effect. Big Pharma is keen on synthesizing medically active marijuana-like molecules that don't make people high —although it's not obvious why mild euphoric feelings are intrinsically negative for a sick person or a healthy person, for that matter. In ancient Greece, the word euphoria meant "having health," a state of well-being. The euphoric qualities of cannabis, far from being an unwholesome side effect, are deeply implicated in the therapeutic value of the plant.

➢ **CBD is sedating.** Moderate doses of CBD are mildly energizing ("alerting"). But very high doses of CBD may trigger a biphasic effect and can be sleep-promoting. If CBD-rich cannabis flower confers a sedating effect, it's likely because of a myrcene-rich terpene profile. Myrcene is a terpene with sedative and painkilling properties. CBD is not intrinsically sedating, but it may help to restore better sleeping patterns by reducing anxiety.

➢ **High doses of CBD work better than than low doses.** CBD isolates require higher doses to be effective than whole plant CBD-rich oil extracts. But that doesn't mean single-molecule CBD is a better therapeutic option than CBD-rich cannabis, which has a wider therapeutic window than a CBD isolate. Reports from clinicians and patients suggest that a synergistic combination of CBD, THC, and other cannabis components can be effective at low doses – as little as 2.5 mg CBD and/or 2.5 mg THC. Some patients may require significantly higher doses of CBD oil to obtain satisfactory results. Keep in mind that CBD and THC and cannabis in general have biphasic properties, meaning that low and high doses can produce opposite effects. An excessive amount of CBD could be less effective therapeutically than a moderate dose.

➢ **CBD converts to THC in a person's stomach.** Orally administered CBD is well-tolerated in humans. But concerns about possible harmful side effects, which might limit CBD's therapeutic utility and market potential, were raised by misleading reports that CBD converts to high-causing THC in the stomach. It does not (read the evidence). There have been extensive clinical trials demonstrating that ingested CBD—even doses above 600 mg—does not cause THC-like psycho-active effects. On the contrary, CBD in sufficient amounts can lessen or neutralize the THC high. The World Health Organization studied the issue and gave CBD a clean bill of health in a 2017 report that asserted: "Simulated gastric fluid does not exactly replicate physiological conditions in the stomach [and] spontaneous conversation of CBD to delta-9-THC has not been demonstrated in humans undergoing CBD treatment."

> **CBD is fully legal in the United States because it's no longer a controlled substance.** Not quite. The 2018 Farm Bill legalized the cultivation of industrial hemp (defined as cannabis with less than 0.3 percent THC) in the United States and removed various derivatives of hemp, including CBD, from the purview of the Drug Enforcement Administration (DEA) and the Controlled Substances Act. But the federal Food and Drug Administration (FDA) views CBD as a pharmaceutical drug. And because it has already approved CBD as a pharmaceutical (Epidiolex) for treating two forms of pediatric epilepsy, the FDA maintains that it is illegal to sell hemp-derived CBD as a dietary supplement. The DEA, meanwhile, retains jurisdiction over CBD derived from marijuana (cannabis with more than 0.3 percent THC), which is still prohibited under federal law. Rooted in reefer madness racism and enforced disproportionately against people

of color, marijuana prohibition is akin to the Confederate statue still standing – a testament to enduring bigotry and social injustice.

➤ **Legalizing CBD, but not cannabis, adequately serves the patient population.** Seventeen U.S. states have enacted "CBD only" (or, better said, "low THC" or "no THC") laws. And 30 states have legalized medical marijuana (not just CBD) in one form or another. Some states restrict the sources of CBD-rich products and specify the diseases for which CBD can be accessed; others do not. But a CBD-rich remedy with little THC doesn't work for everyone. Parents of epileptic children have found that adding some THC (or THCA, the raw, unheated version of THC) helps with seizure control. For some epileptics (and many other people), THC-dominant products are more effective than CBD-rich products. Most patients are not well served by CBD-only laws. They should have access to a broad spectrum of whole plant cannabis remedies, not just low THC medicine. Anything less is a national scandal. One size doesn't fit all with respect to cannabis therapeutics, and neither does one compound or one product or one strain.

➤ **CBD is CBD—It doesn't matter where it comes from.** It may be possible to extract CBD oil from some low-resin industrial hemp cultivars, but fiber hemp is by no means an optimal source of CBD. Industrial hemp typically contains far less cannabidiol than high-resin CBD-rich cannabis flower tops. Huge amounts of industrial hemp are required to extract a small amount of CBD, thereby raising the risk of contaminants because hemp is a "bio-accumulator" that draws toxins from the soil. But the debate over sourcing CBD is quickly becoming moot, as plant breeders focus on developing high-resin cannabis varietals (marijuana) that satisfy the legal criteria for industrial hemp – with THC measuring less than 0.3 percent and CBD levels exceeding 10 percent by dry weight. "Pure" CBD extracted and refined from industrial hemp or synthesized in a lab lacks critical medicinal terpenes and other plant compounds that interact with CBD and THC to enhance their therapeutic benefits

THE CBD CHALLENGE

CBD is a molecule, not a miracle. Many people could benefit significantly from legal access to a wide range of cannabis remedies, not just low-THC or no-THC products. CBD alone may not always do the trick. There is compelling evidence that CBD works best in combination with THC and the full spectrum of other cannabis components.

Figuring out how to optimize one's therapeutic use of cannabis is the driving force behind the great laboratory experiment in democracy known as medical marijuana that's been unfolding state-by-state and country-by-country in recent years.

The advent of potent cannabis oil concentrates, non-intoxicating CBD-rich products, and innovative, smokeless delivery systems has transformed the therapeutic landscape and changed the public conversation about cannabis.

It's no longer a matter of debating whether cannabis has merit as an herbal medication – today the key challenge is discerning how to utilize cannabis for maximum therapeutic benefit. Given its low-risk profile, many people are using CBD as an add-on therapy to their existing treatment plans.

But most health professionals know little about CBD or cannabis therapeutics and they lack sufficient expertise to adequately counsel patients regarding dosage, modes of administration, CBD/THC synergies, and any risk factors, including interactions with other drugs.

Instead, the onus has been on a loose-knit community of

self-reliant patients, supportive families and a few pioneer physicians who've learned a lot through trial and error and shared information about how to navigate promising avenues of cannabis therapy.

QUESTION:

CBD has been tested and approved for one specific use. Does this mean it is safe and will soon have approval for other uses?

ANSWER A:

The research is emerging to support the use of CBD for numerous conditions, as well as looking closely at safety, side effects, and long-term effects.

There are some valid concerns about long-term use that must be tested before CBD can be recommended for other diseases. As one approach to pain management, it is seen as an alternative option to the addicting narcotics.

The use of CBD oil might complement a medical approach to treating physical and mental diseases. It is worth discussing with your doctor.

QUESTION:

Does CBD show up in drug tests?

ANSWER B:

Hemp-derived CBD isn't pot, but depending on the strain it could contain trace amounts of THC — not even close to amounts that will get you high. If you're using extremely high doses of CBD (looking at 1000 mg a day or higher every day), your exposure may be high enough to give you a positive result. This should be considered a false positive result, since CBD use is not drug use. But, interpretation is up to the party who orders the test.

If your employer does random drug screens, dig into your HR materials to see if using CBD might lead to any hassle.

CHAPTER 9

CBD oil

CBD oil is made by extracting resin from the stalks of hemp or cannabis flowers and then diluting it with a carrier oil such as coconut or olive oil. Most of the CBD oil used for medicinal purposes comes from hemp.

Both scientific studies and anecdotal evidence reveal that CBD oil is helpful in reducing the symptoms of a wide variety of ailments. Although some of the health issues may differ, recent studies have shown that the body's endocannabinoid system is the common thread. Named after the cannabis plant, the endocannabinoid system consists of receptors & molecules that inhabit the brain, organs, glands, and cells within the human body.

The endocannabinoid system performs different jobs in various parts of the central nervous system with the overarching goal of creating a stable equilibrium throughout the human body. The balance that the endocannabinoid system maintains between tissues, organs, and cells enables the body's systems to perform at peak performance.

Most commonly, you'll see CBD oil infused in extra virgin olive oil. This involves steeping the plant in olive oil for several weeks. If you need it now, you can buy CBD infused oil, or if you can get your hands on some high-CBD plant material, you can extract your own. CBD infused oils are perishable, so keep it in a dark glass container in the fridge.

HOW TO USE CBD OIL FOR PAIN RELIEF

Phytocannabinoids occur naturally in cannabis plants. There are fifteen subclasses of such compounds. THC, cannabidiol, and cannabidivarin are some examples of the same. Cannabidiol (CBD) is a subclass of Phytocannabinoids and one among one twenty cannabis compounds. It is hailed for its ability to be meditative, without causing a euphoric high. This non-addictive miracle cannabinoid has been the talk of the town and the core of numerous experiments. The anti-inflammatory properties of CBD have inspired the marketing of its by-products, such as CBD oil, for pain relief and relaxation

THE HEALTH BENEFITS OF CBD OIL

Epilepsy

Cannabidiol has been widely accepted as an anti-psychotic family member of the cannabis family. Ongoing studies have involved inspecting the use of CBD in helping victims of Post-Traumatic Stress Disorder.

CBD oil has definitely proven to subdue symptoms of anxiety, to the extent that the US Food and Drug Administration has approved the use of Epidilolex, a patented CBD medicine, for the treatment of epilepsy and the repetitive seizures induced by the affliction. Similarly, CBD oil can be effective in the treatment of stress-related bodily ailments.

MULTIPLE SCLEROSIS

Multiple Sclerosis is a condition in which the immune system mistakenly reacts abhorrently to healthy cells and organs. Also known as an autoimmune disease, multiple sclerosis causes reoccurring spasms and enduring pain, for those affected. Although the effect is modest, CBD oil, acting as an anticonvulsant, can help in mitigating the number of spasms caused, as well as the resulting pain.

ARTHRITICS

One of the most profound uses of cannabidiol oil is for the relief of arthritic pain. There are two kinds of arthritis, rheumatoid and osteoarthritis, both resulting in swelling and stiffness in joints. Scientific studies have documented that the application of CBD oil can help assuage the pain caused by inflammations. Results have been encouraging. Health associations and the government, alike, are optimistic about the role of CBD oil in bringing solace to arthritic patients.

AUTISM

Of the many developmental disorders, autism and its associated spectrum of disorders are perhaps the most pervasive. Autistic children suffer from insomnia, irritability and a loss of appetite, to name a few. Practitioners have been experimenting with the use of CBD oil in curtailing the social anxiety and psychological manifestations vicariously caused in victims of autism.

A paper by Cassuto and Lubotzky documented the reduction in the number of behavior outbreaks in autistic children treated with medical cannabis, particularly Cannabidiol. Similarly, anxiety and communication problems were mitigated. Hence, CBD oil could have a future in the treatment of the symptoms of autism spectrum disorders.

CRAMPS, CHRONIC PAIN, AND ADDICTION

There have been a number of studies investigating the conceivable part of CBD oil in vanquishing pain of all proportions, be it menstrual cramps or pain of a chronic magnitude. The Journal of Experimental medicine speaks about the utilization of CBD oil for suppressing neuropathic pain in rodents. In spite of the fact that such studies are yet to be replicated with human beings, CBD oil is a good tolerance-builder, an agent that enhances the physique's ability to cope with and be resilient to pain.

Furthermore, CBD oil can be called the antithesis of cannabinoids, and help in the cessation of smoking as well as other additions. Scientific research is charting the evidence for the same.

It is clear that CBD oil has a number of functions in pain relief and regulation. However, there are a few arguments that are worth considering. One is the use of CBD oil on children. Although proven to be a player in autism-symptom mitigation, the influence of CBD oil on the developing brain has yet to be deemed unintrusive. It is still not recommended that CBD be used extensively on children. The recommended dosage of CBD oil for children and adults, both, must be determined in consultation with a doctor.

CBD oil might also cause fatigue, diarrhoea and sudden weight gain/weight loss, depending on each individual's ability to metabolise or reaction to the substance. For this reason, it is always important to test the use of CBD oil in limited batches before delving into a long-term treatment program.

Many a time, multiple cannabinoid compounds are used together, either knowingly or unknowingly. It is, hence, tough to discern the extent to which each compound is involved in causing the desired effect. There are cases where a group of cannabinoids works synergistically in bringing about bodily reactions. Studies selectively employing CBD oil are few in number, but promising.

To conclude, the increasing use of CBD oil as a therapeutic substance has inspired many applications. However, caution must be exercised when choosing CBD as a wholesome alternative to allopathic medicine for pain

10 THINGS YOU NEED TO KNOW BEFORE YOU BUY CBD OIL

Many people are now discovering the benefits of CBD oil. CBD is a cannabinoid which is basically chemicals found in the cannabis plant. Some of these cannabinoids contain traces of oil.

One of the most well-known compounds of the cannabis plant is THC or tetrahydrocannabinol. Once the THC is broken down by heat and ingested, it can create a high. Although THC and CBD both come from the cannabis plant, it is only THC which is mind altering and gives you a high.

Although more people are becoming aware of the health benefits of CBD oil, many still associate it with marijuana and getting high. Some of the many known health benefits of CBD oil include pain relief, reducing inflammation, anti-acne, and an antidepressant.

CBD is typically extracted from the cannabis plant as an oil or a powder. The oil or powder can then be mixed with a gel or cream that can be rubbed onto the skin or ingested orally. For first time buyers of CBD oil, it can be a bit of a challenge, as there are many things to consider as CBD oil can come in many different forms. There is also a vast number of different products and brands on the market.

In order to get the CBD oil that best suits your needs, the two most important things to consider are the strength and concentration. Other factors to consider include purity and the volume of CBD oil within the product itself.

Cannabidiol (CBD) oil has become increasingly popular as a natural way to help people try to manage pain, reduce inflammation, and cope with anxiety. Although, the number of prescriptions has risen sharply in the United States over the past 20 years, many Americans are trying to limit the number of prescribed drugs they take – instead, searching for all-natural solutions to the aches, pains, and discomfort they begin to face as they age. For many of them, CBD oil is the solution they've been looking for. But not all CBD oil is created equal, meaning finding the right CBD oil could just be the most important part of their journey.

1. WHERE WAS THE HEMP GROWN AND WHAT MIGHT BE IN IT?

Hemp is a bioaccumulator, meaning it is capable of absorbing both the good and the bad from the air, water, and soil in which it's grown. This makes it all the more important to know that your CBD oil comes from organically grown hemp that can be tracked to its US-grown source. The last thing buyers want is for their CBD oil to have accumulated toxic substances such as pesticides, herbicides, or heavy metals. For decades, farmers have used pesticides to protect crops against insects, disease, and fungi – and have used herbicides to control weeds – but we've known for quite some time that chemicals used to harm other species can also be harmful to our own species. That's one big reason behind the global push to go organic. People are starting to prioritize organic crops, whether you're talking about fruits, vegetables, grains, legumes, nuts, livestock feed – even textiles like cotton, wool, and flax.

Types of Cancer Linked to Pesticides/Herbicides

- Leukemia
- Non-Hodgkin lymphoma
- Multiple myeloma

- Soft tissue sarcoma
- Cancers of the skin, lip, stomach, brain, prostate

Due to the potential dangers of these chemicals, the list of organic products people should seek out absolutely includes hemp – and the only way you can be sure that the CBD oil you buy is pure and free of foreign substances is by purchasing CBD oil from an organic source that can be traced all the way back to the field.

Key Factors in Sourcing

- Organically grown
- Grown in the United States
- Transparent seller

2. HOW MUCH THC IS IN THE CBD OIL?

For some, having more than trace amounts of Tetrahy-drocannabinol (THC) might not be a big deal, but if you're being drug tested at work, operating heavy machinery, or fall into a number of other categories, you may want to keep the THC to a bare minimum. In order to qualify as a legal hemp product, CBD oil must contain less than 0.03% THC. Look for CBD oil certified to have low levels of, or zero, THC in them. Many reputable sellers do offer products that have absolutely no THC in them at all, so if you are concerned about keeping even trace amounts of TCH out of your body, it is best to look for those products and sellers.

Benefits of CBD with Less Than 0.03% THC:

- No failed drug tests (if zero THC)
- No fear of mind-altering affects
- Complies with the guidelines of the Substance Abuse and Mental Health Services Administration (SAMHSA)

3. WHAT'S THE CONCENTRATION OF CBD IN THE PRODUCT?

CBD oil is similar to other products in that it is capable of being "watered down." Some companies will try to eke out a higher profit margin by fooling their customers into thinking they're getting more for less. It is important to pay attention to the concentration level of the CBD oil you're buying in order to ensure you're getting what you're paying for. Although concentrations of CBD can vary quite a bit across the broad range of CBD products, a quality product will start off having somewhere between 250mg to 1,000mg per fluid ounce. This matters because if you were to purchase a 4 ounce bottle that contained 250mg of CBD, your concentration would be a mere 62.5 mg of CBD per ounce – hardly enough to reap the full benefits of CBD. It's always important to look at the concentration level of the CBD you're buying.

If the concentration of CBD is not listed, use the following formula to help guide your purchase:

Total amount of CBD (in mg)/volume of container (in ounces) = concentration level

Example: 1,500mg CBD/4 ounce bottle = 375mg/oz.

4. HOW DO WE KNOW THE CBD IS POTENT AND PURE?

Death and taxes are the only guarantees we have in life, so it's important not to just take a company's word for it that their CBD oil is free of contaminants. Having the CBD tested in a third-party accredited laboratory, free of the watchful eye of the company president, is the only way to ensure the safety, quality, and potency of the product.

Accredited Laboratories Should Test to Ensure the CBD is Free Of:

- Pesticides
- Residual solvents (from the extraction process)
- Bacteria and fungus
- Foreign matter
- Heavy metals

5. HOW MUCH TOTAL CBD IS IN THE PRODUCT?

This may seem like a repeat of an earlier question, but while that question related to concentration of CBD in the product, this is simply a question of how much you're getting in total. Most bottles are labeled in a similar way – "1,000mg CBD Oil" or "1,000mg Hemp Extract" – which generally means the entire bottle contains a total of 1,000mg of CBD.

6. HOW IS THE CBD BEING EXTRACTED?

To get almonds from an almond tree, you can just shake the tree. To get juice from an orange, you can simply squeeze the fruit. But getting CBD oil from hemp is a much more complicated process. The cheapest and easiest ways to extract CBD oil from hemp commonly involve harsh solvents that can leave chemical residue in the CBD oil. The best, and most reliable extraction method, uses carbon dioxide (CO_2) under high pressure and extremely low temperatures to pull out as much CBD as possible without introducing contaminants. Once the CO_2 is no longer under intense pressure, it simply evaporates, leaving virtually no trace of extraction on the CBD oil.

Benefits of CO2 Extraction:

- Ensures high quality
- Uses no harsh solvents/chemicals
- Free of butane & propane, and ethanol
- It's a standard solvent, widely used for foods and dietary supplements

7. IS THERE ANY ACCOUNTABILITY?

Some companies will hide under a cloak of darkness that the Internet can provide, but it's a pretty good sign if the company lists an honest-to-goodness phone number you can use to reach real people. The companies with inferior products will often be very difficult to reach. Before ordering, try to reach out to the company. If someone picks up the phone or gets back to you in a timely manner, you've probably found a company that not only takes accountability seriously, but cares about their customers and the quality of their products.

8. IS THE COMPANY HIDING SOMETHING?

It's important to search for CBD products that are sold legally, with full transparency and accountability. There are myriad shady businesses, false claims, and products of inferior quality in the supplement industry. Finding a transparent CBD company is the first step to finding an ethical CBD company.

9. WHAT ARE THEY CLAIMING?

It is a strict violation of the Food and Drug Administration DSHEA guidelines to make medical claims about the efficacy of CBD products in the treatment of any medical condition or symptom. Although preliminary research has shown tremendous promise of CBD oil helping people in pretty remarkable ways, legitimate CBD companies will refrain from making any direct medical claims. Be very wary of companies that defy this guideline, because if they disregard this particular rule, what other rules are they willing to ignore?

10. IS CHEAPER ALWAYS BETTER?

When it comes to CBD oil, cheaper is most certainly not always better because the production of quality CBD oil just isn't cheap. CO_2 extraction utilizes complex equipment and a high level of expertise as opposed to the cheaper and easier chemical extraction processes that can leave residue from toxic solvents like butane, propane, and ethanol in the CBD oil. While the CO_2 extraction will generally lead to a higher price tag, it does insure quality, purity, and potency –especially when used to extract CBD oil from hemp that has been organically grown in the United States.

Reasons Higher-Quality CBD Oil May Cost More

- Organically grown
- Extracted using CO_2 method
- Higher concentrations of CBD
- Grown in the United States
- Tested in third-party labs
- Company is following rules/laws
- Made from high-quality, full-spectrum extract, so other beneficial compounds are present.

HOW TO USE CBD OIL

CBD is just one of many compounds in marijuana, and it is not psychoactive. Smoking cannabis is not the same as using CBD oil. Using CBD oil is not the same as using or smoking whole cannabis. A person can use CBD oil in different ways to relieve various symptoms. If a doctor prescribes it to treat LGS or DS, it is important to follow their instructions.

CBD-based products come in many forms. Some can be mixed into different foods or drinks or taken with a pipette or dropper. Others are available in capsules or as a thick paste to be massaged into the skin. Some products are available as sprays to be administered under the tongue. Recommended dosages vary between individuals, and depend on factors such as body weight, the concentration of the product, and the health issue.

Due to the lack of FDA regulation for most CBD products, seek advice from a medical professional before determining the best dosage. As regulation in the U.S. increases, more specific dosages and prescriptions will start to emerge. After discussing dosages and risks with a doctor, and researching regional local laws, it is important to compare different brands of CBD oil.

There is a selection of CBD products available for purchase online.

HOW TO MAKE CBD OIL IN 5 STEPS

1. **Check your state laws.** Making CBD oil requires possession of cannabis plant material, which is a controlled substance. So, do a little CYA and find out what's allowed and what could get you into trouble. Don't skip this part!
2. **Source your plant material.** You need a good amount of dried buds of a high-CBD strain of cannabis that has only trace amounts of THC if any.
3. **Decarboxylate.** Sounds like something out of a science lab, but this just means you spread them out on a baking sheet and bake them for 45 minutes at 225. This step makes the medicinal oils in the plant more bioavailable.
4. **Steep.** Transfer your buds to a glass jar, leaving a little room at the top. Completely cover the buds with lightweight oils like extra virgin olive oil or sweet almond oil. Put a lid on and let them sit for 2-3 weeks. A couple times per week throughout the steeping process, you should flip the jar over and back upright to distribute the oil.
5. **Strain.** Use a cheesecloth-lined strainer to separate all the plant material from the oil. Now you have CBD infused oil to use as-is or to make into salves and balms. There are lots of recipes online for that. Store it in a dark glass container in the fridge.

If your oil takes on a funky smell or grows scum or fuzz at any point during or after the process, dump it into the trash and start over.

CBD OIL VS HEMP OIL VS CANNABIS SATIVA VS CANNABIS OIL: A CLEAR DESCRIPTION OF EACH, AND THEIR USES

Cannabis Sativa is the botanical name of the plant species. There are multiple strains of the Cannabis Sativa plant. One of the common strains is called Industrial Hemp which is where the Hemp Oil and CBD Oil are derived, and the other is Marijuana. These are different plants, but both come from the same family of plants. Industrial Hemp naturally produces higher levels of Cannabidiols (CBD) and low levels of tetrahydrocannabinol (THC).

Industrial Hemp has been legalized for cultivating in the USA according to the Farm Bill Act and is where most Hemp Oil and CBD Oil products come from. Marijuana plants are just the opposite producing high levels of THC and lower levels of CBD. The legal status of Marijuana varies vastly from state to state.

CBD Oil or Hemp Extract- CBD Oil, often times referred to as Hemp Extract. Hemp extract is an extract with naturally occurring terpenes, flavonoids, Cannabinoids, and other beneficial phytonutrients from the hemp plant. This CO_2 extracted Hemp oil or CBD Oil is free of harmful solvents and uses a gentle, low temperature, alcohol free extraction process that yields the purest form of Hemp oil extract or CBD Oil available. This clean oil extraction process yields a high quality extracted hemp oil retaining a broad spectrum of terpenes, Cannabinoids, and other phyto-compounds derived from the Cannabis Sativa industrial hemp plant like CBD Oil. CBD Oil is most commonly used to assist with Pain, Stress, Anxiety, Sleep, Inflammation, etc. This is due to the Cannabinoids present.

Hemp Oil is most commonly sourced from the Cannabis Sativa (Industrial Hemp) plant seed. It is also called Hemp Oil or Hemp Seed Oil. Hemp Oil is regulated in its production and is tested for THC and CBD levels, however it does not contain either of those Cannabinoids. Test have shown that there are no cannabinoids present in the seeds of the hemp plant. Hemp Oil is most commonly referred to as a Superfood, because of the high levels of Omegas, Vitamins, and other Nutrients. It may also assist with Pain, and stress due to its naturally occurring nutrients. Hemp Oil is also excellent for Hair and skin thanks to all of those Omegas and Vitamins!

Cannabis Oil is commonly from the marijuana plant but can vary depending on the manufacturer as Cannabis is also the botanical name of the Industrial Hemp plant. The Cannabis oil from the Marijuana strain is extracted from the Marijuana plant. It contains high levels of THC and lower levels of CBD Oil. Cannabis Oil from the Marijuana plant is illegal in most states. It is used for medicinal purposes and as a recreational drug. It is not regulated in its production.

www.ingramcontent.com/pod-product-compliance
Lightning Source LLC
Chambersburg PA
CBHW030627220526
45463CB00004B/1437